Is Weight Loss Surgery
Right For You?

Is Weight Loss Surgery
Right For You?

◆

Eight Stories to Help You Decide

Glenn Goldberg

iUniverse, Inc.

New York Lincoln Shanghai

Is Weight Loss Surgery Right For You?
Eight Stories to Help You Decide

iUniverse books may be ordered through booksellers or by contacting:

iUniverse
2021 Pine Lake Road, Suite 100
Lincoln, NE 68512
www.iuniverse.com
1-800-Authors (1-800-288-4677)

ISBN-13: 978-0-595-37968-2 (pbk)
ISBN-13: 978-0-595-82337-6 (ebk)
ISBN-10: 0-595-37968-0 (pbk)
ISBN-10: 0-595-82337-8 (ebk)

Printed in the United States of America

To Jesse Goldberg, our beloved daughter—

She makes every second of life worthwhile.

Contents

Introduction

**This is the book that I desperately needed—but that didn't exist—
when I struggled to decide whether I really wanted to
surgically make my stomach the size of my thumb.**

This book shares my feelings, insights, and perspectives as I moved along my personal path to and from *weight loss surgery* (WLS). I have now used the WLS tool to remedy my morbid obesity, repair my health, ease my suffering, and prolong my life.

In the two years since my surgery, I've lost half of my starting weight of 360 pounds. Today, I'm stabilized at my ideal weight of 180 pounds, so I'm "half the man" I used to be. I look and feel great. I savor every minute of my priceless second chance to live a long, active, and healthful life.

However, I still remember the dark fears and deep skepticism that fueled my reluctance to *even consider* this drastic, expensive surgery of "last resort." I felt desperately alone, confused, and overwhelmed. I felt ashamed that I couldn't lose my excess weight the "normal way," by dieting and exercise. I had so many difficult questions demanding straightforward and honest answers, but I didn't know whom to ask or trust. I was scared about the risks, and urgently needed to know what to expect—physically, emotionally, socially, and financially. I had heard horror stories about "gastric bypass gone bad." Therefore, I resisted trying, or even considering, what might be the latest in a long series of costly, dangerous fads, extreme diets, and false solutions. I honestly didn't think that I could handle another failure.

I feared that, even with the surgery, I would sabotage myself with my binges and my out-of-control compulsive overeating that had put on the pounds and evaded any solutions. I didn't know where to start or how to proceed. Nevertheless, I did my best to make an informed choice that was right for me.

I surfed the Web, scanned Web sites, devoured WLS books, joined WLS patient e-mail groups, and met with several postoperative patients. I attended my bariatric surgeon's informational orientation and peppered him with my questions. My choice became clear. I started down the WLS path.

And yet, after undergoing the procedure, I found myself disappointed, angry, and resentful. Not because I was unhappy with the outcome; I'm thrilled with my results and satisfied with the trade-offs. I was upset because—despite my careful and systematic inquiries—I had no idea how difficult and challenging it would be to succeed and thrive after WLS. I felt "ripped off," misled, and deceived by the illusions or delusions created by my pre-op explorations.

In the clarity of hindsight, I now suspect that many of the WLS patients whose sharing I relied upon had unconsciously sugar coated their postoperative accounts. I know now, from personal experience, that after I had lost my excess weight and survived the ordeal, many of the worst aspects and challenges seemed to fade from my memory and awareness. Perhaps this is similar to how a woman may subconsciously repress some or much of her pain and difficulty after she's recovered from childbirth.

Whatever the reason, I decided, right then and there, that I would do everything in my power to ensure that people making the WLS decision had a full, fair, and fearlessly honest and balanced understanding (the good, the bad, and the ugly) of the implications and consequences of their choice. My intent was not to encourage or discourage people from choosing WLS. Rather, I wanted to ensure that they have the truth, and nothing but the truth, about the option and experience, at the outset, to help them make choices that are right for them.

I created a Web site (www.weightlosssurgerycoach.com) and started journaling and disseminating my newsletter (titled "**Through Thick** and Thin"), once I decided to have the surgery (about four months before my operation). I've continued writing my newsletter and sharing my experiences and challenges with many thousands of WLS-ers throughout my first two years post-op.

When I started my newsletter chronicling my WLS experience, I had two positive intentions. The first was selfless—to share my trials, encouragement, and hope with others journeying along the same path. The second was quite selfish—to reinforce my commitment and to avoid sabotaging myself the way I had for several decades of compulsive overeating, obsessive dieting, gluttony, and shame. I figured that by going public with my decision and progress, I would turn my tendency to blame myself into a positive tool that would help me avoid the humiliation, defeat, and disaster of backsliding and failing yet again.

I'm celebrating my second anniversary of my weight loss surgery by publishing this anthology. It begins with my own story. Chapter 1 describes my decision-making process and preparations for surgery, and it ends with my being wheeled into the operating room, prepared to die and praying for life. Chapter 2 chronicles my surgery experience and postoperative challenges, surprises, and successes.

Chapter 3 documents my transformation from *fat* to *fit*—living in a "normal-sized" body, no longer defined or limited by obesity. Chapter 4 presents my bottom lines—my overall assessment, two years out from my surgery: what I've gained, what I've given up, and my trade-offs and conclusions.

Issues of my newsletter, which are published in this book, enable the reader to vicariously share all aspects of my WLS experience as it has unfolded. My writings explore the origins of my obesity, my WLS decision-making process, my preoperative preparations, and my postoperative recovery. The newsletters present the most honest overview I can offer of my physical, emotional, and lifestyle transformation.

My story is followed by much briefer stories of seven other WLS patients—very different tales from very different people—but all featuring the same kind of honesty, balance, and emotional insights I strive to share. I'm sure that every reader will be able to relate to one or more of the unique perspectives presented. Common themes will emerge. Taken together, these stories underscore what I believe is essential for readers to understand and consider as they move toward making their own WLS decision.

I am not affiliated with any bariatric surgeon, clinic, or hospital. I have no attachment to whatever decision you make. My sole objective is to give you a balanced picture of weight loss surgery so that *whatever* decision you make, you'll know what to expect, and your choice will be fully informed.

PART I

One Man's Thoughts about Weight Loss Surgery

1

Making My
WLS Decision

Through Thick & Thin #1
(Before the Surgery—4 Months)

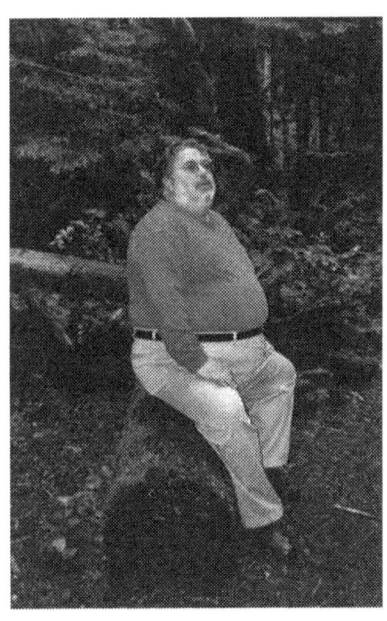

As far back as I can remember, my weight has been a defining, limiting, painful, and self-destructive issue in my life. Today, as I approach age fifty-five and a "morbidly obese" (life-threatening) 360 pounds, I am preparing to have some form of the gastric bypass surgery in four months.

Why am I now choosing to surgically make my stomach the size of my thumb?

It's because I'm *morbidly obese*. How I hate those words and that characterization! However, they accurately and fairly describe at least the physical dimension of who I have become. At 360 pounds, I weigh about 180 pounds more than that "ideal weight" set forth on those damnable charts. And my weight is now becoming a life-threatening condition. As my physical therapist responded when I asked for his advice about having this operation, "How many fat, *old* people do you see around?"

Largely as a product of my weight, I am now an insulin-dependent Type 2 (adult onset) diabetic. I inject myself with insulin before breakfast and dinner and test my blood sugar levels throughout the day. I have obstructive sleep apnea, which requires that I sleep with a mask connected to a continuous positive air pressure (CPAP) apparatus, which forces ambient air down my throat with sufficient

3

pressure to keep the passageway open, and thus keep me breathing and my heart beating. These are considered comorbid conditions—associated with my morbid obesity and, ultimately, also threatening to my health and extended life.

I live with extreme daily pain. I have experienced what seems to be a never-ending series of painful conditions—chronic lower back pain, pinched nerves in my legs, diabetic neuropathy, strained forearms, sore knees, etc. All these conditions—and my discomfort and pain—are ultimately due to my excess weight.

And yet I didn't make the decision to have the gastric bypass surgery merely because I'm tired of the pinpricks, insulin injections, sleeping with a mask and machine, or chronic daily pain. I most assuredly did not decide to have this surgery because of concerns about my appearance or other people's judgments about me or my weight.

Decades ago I began dealing with the painful emotional wounds and demons that drove me to compulsive overeating. Back then, I cast off my feelings of guilt, shame, and blame for my weight and found a measure of self-acceptance and love for the human being I am. And then I became relatively indifferent to the stares, the rude comments, and the judgments of others who saw only hundreds of pounds of accumulated fat, not the extraordinary being hidden and suffering within that insulation.

I made the decision to have weight loss surgery for only one reason—so that I could live a long, healthy, and productive life.

I want more years to be with Kari, my precious and beloved wife and life partner. I want to see my brilliant, talented, and beautiful daughter create an awesome life, career, and family of her own. I want to harvest the fruits of my creative spirit, which become deeper and richer as I age. Ultimately, I made the decision because I have finally admitted to myself that I no longer have any realistic hope or prospect of reducing my morbid obesity "the normal way"—through eating well and exercising.

After I was diagnosed as a diabetic several years ago, I met with a dietician to learn what I needed to understand to take better care of myself. Since then, I have substantially reduced, or stopped completely, my consumption of sugar products, most refined starches, salt, and junk foods. Today I eat well, and with moderation, and usually snack only on fruit or vegetables after dinner. I eat a careful, reasonably prudent selection of healthful foods. I also exercise daily, at least until my various aches, pains, and pinched nerves literally stop me in my tracks. And yet my weight has never lessened in any significant way.

It staggered me a few months ago when my weight grew to be, literally, off the scale. The scale in my doctor's office measures up to 350 pounds, and when my weight exceeded even that maximum, I knew that my situation was truly desperate. I was rudely slapped in the face with the reality that there is no upward limit to my potential for obesity. I have now surrendered hope of this situation ever changing.

So finally, once and for all, I have stopped believing the stories I've been telling myself for most of my life—that eventually, some day, some way, I would find the key to weight loss and its maintenance. I stopped believing my myth that I would once again be able to fit into those outgrown clothes that I have so optimistically stored in boxes in my closet over the last several decades.

Once I decided that the "horse" I had been riding all these years (hoping, wishing, and praying for some magical reduction in my obesity) was finally and irrevocably dead, I got off that illusionary mount that had carried me through the years. And when I did, I was surprised to see and acknowledge the true costs I've incurred in carrying the weight of two or three normal-size people.

I have become accustomed to, and accepting of, an outrageous daily toll of inconvenience, limitation, humiliation, pain, discomfort, and exclusion that no longer feels acceptable to me. So long as I clung to the hope that someday, somehow, I would shed my excess weight, I sincerely believed that my only practical choice was serene acceptance and making the best of a difficult situation. However, now that I truly believe that bariatric (weight loss) surgery will enable me to lose the weight and live longer, I can hardly wait to end the torture in all its nefarious forms, which include:

- Squeezing into transport, concert, or movie seats, classroom desks, or restaurant booths designed for normal-size people

- Struggling to find a comfortable and workable way to stand, sit, or lie; to get down or get up; or to put on my socks, tie my shoes, clip my toenails, scratch my back, or even wipe my behind

- Striving to fit into shirts, pants, and jackets that only yesterday seemed to be unbelievably huge

These simple, basic life tasks have become major life challenges, and they have multiplied my dependency upon loved ones. I hate that, and I'm humiliated by it. My body becomes more rigid, moves slower and slower, less and less, and I can feel it beginning to die a slow and agonizing death.

I say these things not to portray myself as a victim, but to honestly and accurately describe the condition in which I find myself today. I also want to present the context in which I have made the decision to have some form of gastric bypass surgery.

I find myself living mostly in my mind, my heart, and my spirit these days, and these places are vital; fully alive; and overflowing with creativity, understanding, compassion, and love. At the same time, I can feel myself quite literally abandoning my body.

No more. I'm taking my body back. I'm moving back in. And now my decision is fueled and reinforced by more than just my desire to live longer. Now, I want to be comfortable and happy too, not just healthy.

Through Thick and Thin #2
(Before the Surgery—3 Months)

The Origins of My Obesity

As I've reconstructed my long and winding path to morbid obesity, I've made some observations that have surprised and intrigued me. As a child, adolescent, and even young adult, I was never as obese as I thought I was, or as I was told I was. Sure, I was always a husky size when my mother led me through the excruciating annual exercise in humiliation to buy clothes for the new school year. And I was always one of the larger kids in my class.

But my "weight problem" wasn't much of a real problem until I responded to years of relentless blaming, shaming, judging, and criticizing by internalizing the distorted perception that I wasn't "good enough," or worthy of respect, dignity, or love because I weighed too much and my body was huge and repulsive.

When I graduated high school I weighed around 200 pounds (I'm 5'10" tall), and throughout college my weight ranged between 200 and 230. When I look back now at my photographs as a child, teen, and young man, I marvel at how relatively normal I looked. How I felt and saw myself was an altogether different matter: enormous, disgusting, and bloated—like a beached whale rotting on the shore. And then, in a terrible paradox, my distorted negative self-perception drove me to eat compulsively until I became exactly what I feared—even more obese than my self-image.

My weight was the subject of a bitter, ruthless, and never-ending war between my mother and me. She passed away several years ago, tragically and prematurely. I'm grateful that before she died we were able to reach a place of mutual understanding, respect, and appreciation. I was able to accept that her words and actions, however hurtful they may have felt, came from her sincere desire that I be healthy and well. She was able to accept that—notwithstanding my obesity—I was a loving and good man, husband, father, and professional.

But during my childhood, and especially my adolescence, my mom seemed to take personal responsibility for my weight, and for whipping me into acceptable shape. It felt like it was a moral crusade for her. I remember her words, looks, and actions—laden with the harsh and critical overtones of guilt, shame, and blame—trying to convince, coerce, or humiliate me into compliance with her latest proposed diet or plan. I knew that overt resistance was futile, so I became a covert eater—raiding the refrigerator late at night when everyone in the house was asleep. If no one saw me eating, then it didn't count, the calories weren't real, and my weight gain was an illusion.

Looking back, the only way that I felt I could be myself or stand up for myself was by my defiance in continuing to stuff food into my mouth. This was part of a doomed attempt to try to fill the emotional, spiritual hole that I felt deep within me. But this was the "hole of not being enough," and there wasn't enough food in the world to fill it. So I ate compulsively, and for so many reasons.

At first I ate for revenge, or out of defiance, and to achieve a sense of power in my adolescent "dance of independence" with my mom. I stuffed my face out of a sense of shame for lacking the self-respect, self-discipline, and strength to stop my self-destruction. I ate for comfort, for solace, for celebration, or for an escape from boredom.

Unfortunately, by the time I learned how to fill the hole, and meet my emotional needs through self-love and the love of others, I had developed a lifestyle and an array of self-destructive habits that persisted even when the emotional needs that had prompted them were resolved. It's so sad and regrettable. This was a time in my life when some understanding and support, some education about healthful eating, and a reasonable exercise program would have been enough to solve my weight problem. Instead, concerns over my weight inspired verbal and emotional attacks that backfired and yielded counterproductive reactions that turned a potential problem into a serious lifelong health crisis.

My weight became the central aspect of my relationship with my parents. It dominated every phone call and visit. I remember proudly bringing my wife and newborn child to Florida, where my parents had retired, to show them off. I hoped and ached to finally get some measure of approval for becoming a successful man, husband, and father—good enough and worthy of acceptance and respect. And I will never ever forget my intense pain and despair upon entering their home when my mother took a horrified look at my bulk and said, "If I were you, and had to look at that fat face in the mirror every morning, I would just puke."

It hurt me beyond description to know that she saw me as a 280-pound sack of nauseating fat, and nothing more. It devastated my spirit to see that my own mother continued to judge my value as a man by my weight on the scale.

Every interaction with my parents ended the same way: with a bitter, desperate, and unsuccessful effort by my mother to blame and shame me—or later, my wife—into doing what had to be done for me to become a normal, and therefore acceptably sized, human being.

Over the years, I tried every diet, fad, and program. During my early high school years, my mom brought me to a diet doctor who gave me pills and injections guaranteed to solve my problem. Over the course of six months, I lost fifteen pounds, and gained back twenty-five pounds after I stopped seeing him because of the uncomfortable side effects. (I didn't know then that he was prescribing amphetamines to suppress my appetite.)

Next, during summer break from college, I joined Weight Watchers. I continued this program off and on for a few years. I lost twenty pounds, and regained thirty after leaving the program. I hated the weigh-ins, and measuring food and intake, and ultimately rebelled against the regulation and attention to detail, which didn't fit well with my life as an undergraduate. Then I continued my "diet dance" with Stillman's, Atkins's, the grapefruit diet, and so many more. Back and forth to Weight Watchers, and then liquid protein diets, which worked great, until I returned to eating solid foods. Nothing ever worked or lasted.

My appetite regulator never seemed to work right. I never felt full. So I grazed from the time I got up in the morning until the time I fell asleep at night. I weighed 240 pounds when I married Kari in 1979. Our first daughter, Julya, died tragically (and unnecessarily) during her birth because of hospital negligence. Consequently, my eating spiraled out of control, as I unsuccessfully sought solace by eating my way through my unbearable grief. This was a time when people generally didn't acknowledge a still-birth as the loss of a child, which, of course, it was. The death of our child killed all our hopes and dreams for this sweet girl and our future with her. The next year, Kari suffered a late miscarriage, and it was not until our third child was born that we fully recovered that future.

It was only then that I snapped out of my isolation and unconsciousness long enough to weigh myself and found that I had peaked at 350 pounds, and realized—with a feeling of total terror and despair—that there was no upward limit to what I could weigh.

That's when—desperate, scared, and sick with fear and dread—I found my way to Overeaters Anonymous (OA) and their 12-step recovery program. I am forever grateful to OA for the gifts of a belief system, the Serenity Prayer ("God, grant me the serenity to accept the things I cannot change, the courage to change the things I can, and the wisdom to know the difference"), and the fellowship that changed my worldview of life forever.

However, while OA helped me heal my emotional wounds and restore my self-love, self-acceptance, self-pride, and self-respect, my obesity still remained. In the two decades since discovering OA, my food program (and most definitely my attitude and spirituality) has improved. Yet I was never able to make any meaningful or lasting reduction in my obesity.

One of the greatest gifts of OA was my realization that dieting was as dangerous and self-destructive to me as was my compulsive overeating. I resolved to never, ever diet again. Healthful and thoughtful and careful eating programs: fine. But diet: never again!

I also constructed, practiced, and strengthened my emotional boundaries with my parents and other family members. Once I realized that engaging in discussions with my mom about my weight and weight loss strategies was counterproductive—namely, it drove me to eat more and despair more rather than helping in any way—I laid down and enforced the boundaries that *any* discussions of my weight were out of bounds and unacceptable. "If you want to maintain a relationship with me," I told my mom, "you must agree to never talk about my weight."

Of course, she still tried. She tried to enlist my wife as her ally and proxy to manage my weight. When my wife refused to play this game and assume this role, my mother reluctantly stopped talking about it, at least out loud, at least to me. My weight and her concern about it became a popular topic in her discussions with my siblings and other family members. And whenever we visited, I always cringed during that first look-over, during which, however silently, she invariably expressed her disgust.

I know that, from my perspective, both her strategy and her execution were flawed and so very hurtful and counterproductive. I also see that this was what she learned from her mother, and thus the multigenerational cycle of hurt continued to spin. My mother tried to help me the only way she knew how. And now I can forgive, thereby breaking that cycle.

Now, after all these years and all these diets and after the emotional roller coaster ride of my struggles with my weight, I'm finally *ready*. I'm ready to undergo the surgical procedure that I know will deliver the outcome I yearn for, and that my mother always prayed for—my transformation from a morbidly obese man to a man at his ideal and optimally healthful weight.

There are times when I wish I had traveled a different, shorter, and more direct path to this point. Mainly, I'm just grateful that I'm still on this earth, and will soon get my body back. And I'm preparing myself for the dramatic lifestyle, logistical, and emotional changes that will be required for me to successfully complete this transformation. This is not a quick fix, an easy path, or a cure for those weak in spirit and will. I'm ready, and I can't wait to embark.

Through Thick and Thin #3
(Before the Surgery—2.5 Months)

**Jumping Through the Hoops to
Gastric Bypass Surgery**
or
At long last—hope!

For the first time in forty-five years, I truly believe that, through the miracle of this bariatric medical intervention, I can achieve a healthful weight and physical state. Although I have come to feel hopeless about resolving my morbid obesity through careful eating and exercise, I no longer feel helpless.

I've come to realize that I have a serious medical condition that requires a drastic medical intervention. I've accepted that my obesity is not product of deficiencies in my character, intelligence, or competence. There's no shame in that realization. For the first time, I feel hope.

Research indicates that only 5% of dieters are successful, that is, they lose their excess weight and maintain the weight loss. Other research shows that 85% of individuals who have some form of gastric bypass surgery lose at least 40% of their excess weight—and keep it off long term.

I remember reading about the procedure years ago, and fantasizing about it—much like I have fantasized about the discovery of the magic pill that will melt away my unwanted extra pounds, or that will speed up my metabolic rate, or that will otherwise solve my weight problem for me. But I've had a very negative and painful experience with so-called elective surgery, and something that involved stapling my stomach seemed unacceptably bizarre and still too experimental to consider.

This time, however, when I read a *Newsweek* article about the gastric bypass procedure, it seemed that the surgery was now a relatively safe and proven-successful intervention. So I surfed the Internet and checked out the Web sites of the American Society for Bariatric Surgery, Web MD, the *Obesity Surgery Journal*, the Centers for Disease Control and Prevention, ObesityHelp.com, and other similar sites, including several hosted by ecstatic survivors of the procedure. I avidly studied the voluminous information about the surgery at these sites. The more I learned, the more interested and hopeful I became. I also encountered several WLS Web sites and e-mail groups that seemed to emphasize the negative aspects or experiences with the procedure, but I tended to discount them because many of the contributors seemed to be so angry and one-sided in their perspectives about WLS.

Here's what I learned. In 1991, the National Institutes of Health endorsed the procedure as efficacious. Death rates from the surgery remained at a relatively modest rate of about 1.5% (estimates range from 0.5 to 2%, depending on the experience of the bariatric surgeon). The rate of surgical complications seemed to be within a reasonable range (e.g., 5%)—the same as for any major surgery. Patients who had the procedure generally lost their excess weight in rapid and dramatic fashion, and generally kept it off. Often, their diabetes, sleep apnea, and other comorbid conditions disappeared or ameliorated.

So, after discussions with my wife, I decided it was time for us to have a frank heart-to-heart discussion with our trusted family physician. I let him know, when I made the appointment, what I wanted to discuss so that he could be as prepared as possible. I told him at the outset that we wanted straight talk and answers, complete candor, and honesty. How did he assess and compare the risks of this procedure to the potential benefits?

He told us that, from his research and perspective, the risks were minimal, and the potential benefits enormous. My morbid obesity would kill me prematurely, he predicted, one way or another. Along the way, he warned, the extra weight I was carrying around would continue exacting a terrible toll in terms of the daily pain and wear and tear on my muscles, tendons, and joints. Taking off the excess weight would probably prolong my life significantly and prevent a great deal of the painful episodes and conditions. It might even "cure" my diabetes and sleep apnea. From his perspective as my personal physician, the surgery made great sense.

After further discussion, Kari and I agreed. I searched the American Society for Bariatric Surgery Web site to find a highly trained, credentialed, and *experienced* bariatric surgeon in Seattle, the closest big city. I also checked out the surgeon rating feature at ObesityHelp.com, where patients rate their surgeons and bariatric surgery experience.

I chose Dr. James Weber, who has performed *thousands* of gastric bypass procedures, with extremely low rates of fatalities or complications. The last thing I wanted was to be a guinea pig for some new practitioner trying to gain on-the-job training in this potentially lucrative and fast-growing surgical specialty.

I called to request an initial consultation. At first I was surprised and disappointed, and then eventually quite pleased, when his receptionist advised me that the doctor preferred to invite me and my wife to a free orientation and question-and-answer session held monthly at his hospital of choice in Seattle.

Within the first minutes of the orientation, I was almost ready to give up and leave. It became immediately clear that this procedure would not be covered by my medical insurance plan. Fees for the primary surgeon and his assistant surgeon would run about $7,500, and the costs of hospitalization for the four days required could bring the total cost as high as $30,000. Even if we had this kind of money available, how could I ever justify spending so much on this "elective" procedure?

Actually, it was pretty easy, once my wife and I had a chance to process the information and talk it through. We had received an inheritance after the death of my parents that was sufficient to pay off our debts. This gift brought us an enormous sense of peace, security, and optimism about our future.

And yet, what good was all that if I were to die prematurely? What greater or wiser investment could we possibly make than in my health and prolonged life? I am a man of many talents and gifts, and I've never had more exciting creative projects on my desk than now. We quickly decided that there was nothing more important for us than a chance at many, many more years together. My decision was made!

As it turns out, an abdominal ultrasound required by the surgeon as a precondition to the procedure revealed the presence of stones in my gall bladder. Their removal was considered a medically necessary procedure covered by my health plan. Consequently, a portion of the surgery and the hospitalization costs will end up being covered by my insurance. We would have proceeded with the surgery in any event, but were deeply grateful for this blessing in disguise.

Most bariatric surgeons also insist on directing a slow and careful process leading up to the procedure, including an abdominal ultrasound; a psychological evaluation to assure appropriateness for the procedure and the emotional resources to deal with its aftermath; a nutritional evaluation; and sometimes a sleep apnea study, pulmonary function test, and serum cortisol blood test.

I've begun, slowly and carefully, to share my decision with a few family members and friends. Their response has been heartening. After an initial shock and concern about the risks inherent in the surgery, they all offered their total support for anything that would help me to live longer and healthier.

I don't have many fears about the surgery itself. I do have lots of questions about the mechanics of living and eating with a surgically created stomach pouch the size of my thumb. Fortunately, I'm in touch with a few people who have successfully undergone the surgery and are now celebrating its successful outcomes. I plan to question them until all my questions are answered and my anxieties addressed. I'm also starting to check out, and selectively join and monitor, some of the hundreds of WLS patient e-mail groups.

I have purchased and eagerly read WLS books—both by surgeons and patients—to learn everything I can about every aspect of the procedure, recovery, and outcomes.

Occasionally I consider the possibility of dying during the procedure or because of it. More often, I struggle to imagine what I will look like and what I will feel like as the excess weight comes off, and I become more and more comfortable, flexible, and healthful within my body. What will it feel like to be able to move and bend and twist normally again, without constraint or limitation? How will I feel when I look "normal"? What will be the quality of my life when I can function and move without constant pain?

I'm becoming increasingly excited about the Zen of bariatric surgery. Less will be more. Less food will make my stomach feel more full. Food will become a fuel, to be carefully and consistently administered in small, periodic doses. It will no longer be a raging obsession, an enemy, an invader, a killer.

Last weekend, as I enjoyed a regional jazz festival, I noticed a young musician who reminded me of myself as a young man. He was strutting around, resplendent in a tight-fitting black silk shirt, black silk pants, and a gorgeous black blazer. Just for a moment, I saw a glimpse of my future. And it felt so delightfully, joyfully, deliciously good! At long last—hope!

Through Thick and Thin #4
(Before the Surgery—2 Months)

Preparing for My Weight Loss Surgery

Tomorrow is my long-awaited and eagerly anticipated appointment with my doctor to decide which form of weight loss surgery I will have, and to schedule the date. I'm excited, ready, and anxious. Once I decided to have the surgery, I wanted it over and done with *immediately*. Patience has never been one of my character assets. But I've tried to put this mandatory waiting period (a prudent cooling-off period to prevent "buyer's remorse") to good use, by doing what I can to prepare for my gastric bypass—and my blessed deliverance from my dysfunctional appetite regulator.

I've created a Web site (www.weightlosssurgerycoach.com) and my periodic newsletter. I've joined e-mail groups to begin a dialogue with other folks who have had weight loss surgery. There are now enough WLS patients in our small rural community, so I co-created a support group. I've been walking as far as my body and pain permit, on most days of the week. I've continued eating well and with care. But most of all, I've been doing a lot of thinking about this totally new concept of "food as fuel", which I expect will dominate my postsurgery awareness and experience.

I'm totally intrigued, and deeply challenged, by this notion: that with my little, redesigned stomach pouch I'll just be eating food for nutrition, and to sustain and fuel my body, and not for all the other reasons I've always consumed and devoured excessive amounts:

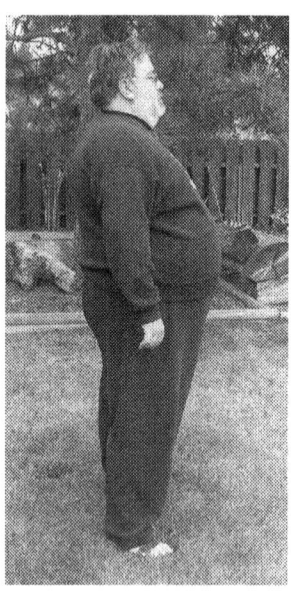

- food for comfort

- food for solace

- food for company

- food for celebration

- food for ups or downs

- food for the kinetic experience and satisfactions

- food to quench my insatiable appetite and fill my bottomless emotional pit

- food to stop the emotional pain

- food to literally stop the hunger pangs

Food has supplied so much of my life's drama, has sometimes played the role of a nurturing mama, and has been the source of so much of my life trauma!

For today, as I look forward to my surgery, I like the idea of leaving this all behind—and of being liberated from the burdens and perils of choice. I like the notion of liquid protein drinks and of eating small, regular portions to fuel my body; of limiting, by gastric necessity, my sugar and fat consumption; of letting go of all the emotional content and connotations of food.

Now, don't get me wrong. I'm a big fan of personal choice. My belief is that I choose my attitude and my frame of reference; that I control what I do with my hands, mouth, and feet; and that I essentially create my own experience and results by the choices I make and the attitudes I choose. But when it comes to food, the abundance of choices can overwhelm, bewilder, bedazzle, and ensnare me. For today, I like the idea of removing food from its traditional emotional context, and just filling up my pouch when and as I need it. I love the concept of leaving my obsessions with tastes and textures behind, along with my outsized body weight.

It feels vital to me to make this mental and emotional switch *before* I have the surgery. Maybe I'll find that this is all nonsense. Maybe I'll find myself yearning for wider choices and for more room in my stomach. But I don't think so.

As I continue to envision a new, thinner, fitter, and healthier me, I'm preparing for my surgery and these outcomes. And, for today, I'm fueled with hope—not overeating.

Through Thick and Thin #5
(Before the Surgery—1.5 Months)

Stuffed in Seattle: Pigging Out and Waking Up
or
There Really Is No Free Lunch

It caught me by surprise one evening last week. I was celebrating a positive meeting with my bariatric surgeon earlier in the day. We had nailed down my late-October surgery date. I was pleased that we had agreed that the vertical banded gastroplasty (VBG) was the best surgical choice for me because this procedure is less drastic and intrusive than the other alternative, with fewer risks of complications. I was also delighted to learn that my VBG won't interfere with my body's natural absorption of nutrients, so I won't require regular vitamin B_{12} injections, and food will flow normally through my stomach. Dr. Weber did not do laparoscopic bands at this time. That surgery was too new for his tried-and-true approach.

I was spending the evening in a hotel room because I had a work assignment in Seattle the next day. I failed to recognize the dangers inherent in breaking my normal meal routine. And so I reverted to old habits and brought snacks, as well as dinner, back to my room. Just in case…

That's when I lost it. And found it. Let me explain: what I lost was my "food sobriety"—my consciousness and awareness of what I had already consumed, how full I was, and when to stop eating. In my complacency, I reverted to old, familiar, but very dangerous ways of thinking (or not) about eating. After an adequate dinner, I continued, throughout the evening, to graze on snack food. I ate after I knew, or at least should have known, that my real hunger was satiated, and that whatever I was feeling came from emotions, and not from hunger. And that's when it hit me: I simply cannot afford *any* lapses *after my surgery.*

This time I got away pretty cheap: an uncomfortable, stuffed feeling, and the guilt of gorging. After my surgery, however, this kind of lapse into eating unconsciousness could jeopardize my surgery, tear out my staples, stretch my stomach pouch, jeopardize my weight loss, and even risk my life. It scared the hell out of me! As well it should. And in the midst of my fear, anxiety, and guilt, I found the gifts and blessings inherent in this episode.

Gifts and blessings? Yes, because the experience gave me an extraordinary opportunity to learn and remember—this time, at least, without the terrible price I could have paid after my surgery. This reversion was a cheap lesson that branded, indelibly, upon my consciousness the admonition that I must remain aware, vigilant, and ready to never, ever fall into that hole again. *This is not a game, an experiment, or a diversion; this is my life that's at stake!*

I set myself up with my own complacency. I do get it now, deep in my gut: there really is no free lunch when it comes to bariatric surgery. The surgery will reduce the size of my stomach pouch, and it will give me the appetite regulator I've always lacked and wanted. It will give me a fair chance to lose the weight. But my eternal vigilance will be the price I must pay to achieve and maintain my health. And it's worth it.

And I'm clear now that each time I fight off the impulse to slide into unconsciousness, my own personal power will be strengthened and multiplied. Every time I resist, I'm gaining power over my addiction.

Now that the lapse is over and done with, I'm grateful that it happened because what it taught me is so much more important than what it cost me. And now, before the surgery, is the time for me to learn this lesson, once and for all, and to steel my resolve. This scary episode of being "stuffed in Seattle" was my last and best chance to look inside and shift my paradigm so that I will never, ever again lapse into eating unconsciousness. I can't afford it. And I will not.

Through Thick and Thin #6
(Before the Surgery—1 Month)

My New Second Job
or
Play Becomes Part of My Lifework

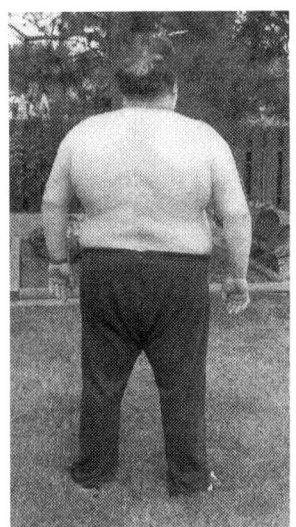

As I continue preparations for my weight loss surgery, I'm learning and accepting that I now must take on a second job—not as part of any new career path. My new job is vigorous daily exercise. It is an absolutely vital precondition to my efforts at reclaiming my body, restoring my health, and prolonging my life. And it's become very clear that unless I perform this job with as much commitment and consistency as all my other work, I will squander my time, money, and this precious opportunity. After all, what meaning will my other lifework have if I don't live long enough to perform it?

For years I've enjoyed a tradition of setting clear, explicit, and challenging goals in every area of my life—personal, family, professional, relationships, and financial—on the first day of each new year. Then, on the next New Year's Eve, I assess my successes and failures. And I've compiled a fantastic track record of meeting, exceeding, or at least approaching all these goals—with one notable exception.

It's the same exception each year. The one that reads something like this: "My health, healthy eating, exercise, and fitness will be vital and integral aspects of my daily life, and balance my professional work. I will feel better and be more fit, weigh less, and experience more freedom and flexibility in movement. My diabetes and sleep apnea will be controlled and will not impair my life or experience. I will exercise on a daily basis." Great sentiments and intentions, but never any follow-through or success. So every New Year's Eve, I wallow in the same pit of frustration, guilt, shame, remorse, humiliation, desperation, hopelessness, and helplessness.

Of course, I always have lots of good reasons, compelling reasons, really, that almost convince me—starting with my chronic body pain and the way that my lower back and legs start to hurt after a quarter-mile and really get in the way after a half-mile—and continuing with the demands of my work and my perfectionism, with earning a living to support my family, and with having enough quality time with my wife, daughter, and friends. Great reasons.

The path to my premature death has been paved with my positive intentions and great excuses and rationalizations.

So when my WLS doctor insisted that I *immediately* begin a daily program of vigorous and sustained exercise in preparation for my WLS, and to promote my weight loss and fitness after it, I was ready with all the explanations of how I was already doing the best I could, and how I would continue, in very good faith, to keep trying. He wasn't buying. And this time, neither was I.

He suggested water aerobics—starting the next day. Well, the next day stretched into a few weeks. And that gave me lots of time to catalogue and document all the excellent reasons why water aerobics wasn't for me. It wouldn't give me as much of a workout as walking. (Wrong. It turns out that my fifty-five-minute workout, given the extra resistance offered by the water, affords me a far greater aerobic workout than walking or other on-land activities.) The participants would be all women, and mostly old women, which was pretty much true, but that's become part of the pleasure of it, and I have the locker room to myself. The music would be awful and the rah-rah spirit depressing. (The music is growing on me, and the instructors have been very kind and don't resemble Richard Simmons at all.) Morning water aerobics would delay the start of my work day and therefore increase my stress. (Wrong again. I feel so much better and more relaxed afterward that I'm now far more productive in far less time.) And it would be too expensive. (At $3 per day, it's far more economical than soda, tobacco, or fast food, and the cost-benefit ratio is extraordinary.)

So I'm now enjoying my second week of daily water aerobics, and I'm feeling great and loving it! Once the endorphins kick in, I experience a wonderful natural high. And what a joy it is to finally jettison that heavy daily burden of guilt and self-loathing that I experienced every day I failed, yet again, to fulfill my commitment to myself. And I've learned some very important lessons:

- That what I most resist is usually exactly what I most need to do

- That taking care of my body, my health, and myself is truly my Job #1

- That if I don't do whatever it takes to lose my excess weight and survive, nothing else—neither my relationships nor my dreams, intentions, goals, projects, and plans—matter much

I'm already looking forward to next New Year's Eve, when for the first time since I started making my list and checking it twice, *every one* of my resolutions will be met! The prospect of breaking this barrier gives me enormous hope that my WLS will empower me to reach my body-health-fitness goal, and that, one day at a time, I can and will do *whatever it takes* to live, healthy and long.

Through Thick and Thin #7
(Before the Surgery—4 Days)

Imagining a Life in Which My Weight Doesn't Run Me As I Pass to the Losing Side

After months of waiting and imagining, my weight loss surgery is just days away. I've been busy completing my work commitments; pursuing emotional closure with family and friends because I don't want to leave anything unsaid, just in case; visualizing my successful surgery and recovery; completing preparations for life post-op by ordering protein powders, planning nutritional choices and an exercise program; and mustering and focusing 100% of my physical, emotional, and spiritual energies on surviving the surgery and emerging on the losing side.

My style is not to immerse myself in my fears and anxieties until I'm on the table, and then to turn my life and this process over to my God, a power greater than myself. And I feel absolutely confident in my doctor and my choice and absolutely confident that my strong body; my powerful heart; my love for my wife, daughter, family, and friends; and a beneficent Universe will get me through to start the rest of my life as a healthy, fit, vigorous man.

I find myself thinking more and more about something one of my e-mail group correspondents noted early in our dialogue. It was a simple statement, and yet it blew me away. It led to the kind of transformative paradigm shift in my worldview that changes *everything* for me. She predicted that there would come a time, within the first two years after my WLS, when my weight would no longer be a primary, defining, or limiting issue in my life—when my obesity would no longer threaten my health, dominate my fears, mass produce my guilt and shame, or top my wish list. Wow!

I have a pretty fertile and resourceful imagination, but imagining this stopped me in my tracks. My mind knows that this is true. My heart continues its skeptical resistance. And, of course, this is precisely the outcome that has led me to pursue this surgery. So I'm going to "act as if" I already believe that this is my future and my destiny, until the day I can drop the act, and live and thrive in the actual reality.

I'm finally ready to undergo the surgery and move to the losing side of weight loss.

2

My Surgical Experience

The Day of My Surgery

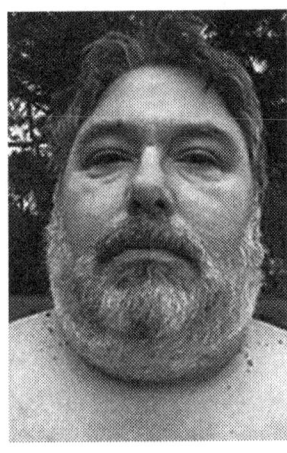

Very early in the morning, a few hours before my alarm would wake me for the short drive from our motel to the hospital for my weight loss surgery, I had a vivid dream.

In the dream, I had been somehow cut up with knives and my body was covered with blood, but I was otherwise unhurt and felt totally comfortable, peaceful, and at ease. I started running—barefoot, effortlessly, and at an astounding speed—along the flat and empty roads. This was an activity and sensation I hadn't experienced in my waking life for many decades due to my obesity and pain-wracked body. I had an unmistakable sense that I was running toward my future.

I encountered several people on this thrilling dream run, and considered asking them for help (as I so often needed to do, in my waking life), until I realized that I really didn't need anyone's help. I was doing just fine on my own and savored the exhilarating sensation of running so fast and so easily. I felt an incredible lightness of being.

Suddenly, in my dream, the scene transformed, and I was a passenger in the backseat of a car driving along a particularly magnificent stretch of highway between the forested mountains towering above and the crashing surf far below. I recognized the road immediately as a stretch near Big Sur, California, close to my former home and one of my most favorite, breathtakingly beautiful spots in the world. Suddenly, and without any apparent reason, I threw open the car door and leaped off the cliff! I soared on the wind currents like an eagle—again effortlessly and without any fear—higher and higher…until I woke up. I awoke feeling an extraordinary sense of safety, health, and well-being.

It was a powerful and reassuring dream to have just before, quite literally, going under the knife. My dream helped me achieve a state of peace and tranquility as I checked into the hospital for my VBG.

At 7:45 that morning, I impatiently waited my turn on the hospital's busy surgical ward. I was feeling ravenously hungry because I had been cautioned to have no food or beverage since the afternoon before, and Kari reminded me, with her usual wonderful sense of humor, that soon I wouldn't be hungry anymore.

As they prepared to roll me into the operating room, my long suppressed fears briefly surfaced. I tend to keep my terror on the shelf until the moment of danger approaches. This was the first moment that I let myself fully feel and acknowledge my fear. My sense of serenity, still lingering from my dream, was superseded by a moment of panic as I kissed Kari goodbye. (What if I died on the table? What if I never saw her again? What if…?)

The night before surgery, I had made a series of phone calls to my family and friends to make sure that nothing was left unsaid, just in case I didn't survive the procedure. My mistake was waiting until literally the last minute to share my fears and tears with my beloved wife and life partner.

The staff wheeled me on a gurney into the operating room. The anesthesiologist administered a sedative, and I don't remember much after that. I do recall that he suggested shaving off my beard so that my oxygen mask would fit better during the surgery. This issue had never been raised before, and I found it to be the worst possible time to discuss it. I wasn't sure if he was joking, but I was very clear and firm, even in my foggy state, that if I was going to die, it would be with my beard intact. That ended the debate. Both my beard and I survived the surgery.

I experienced two other disturbing upsets before going under. The medical staff needed to insert a breathing tube down my unusually small and narrow throat to ensure that, despite my sleep apnea, I would be able to breathe deeply and safely throughout the procedure. Given a real choice (or the availability of Kari to advocate for me), I would have insisted that this tube be inserted *after* I was knocked out. In my confused, sedated state, I endured someone spraying a nauseating local anesthetic down my throat while shoving the breathing tube down my throat passage until I gagged. This was *not* fun. Later, I learned that it would have been no problem, and would have made me much more comfortable, if the tube had been inserted *after* I was fully anesthetized.

I was not prepared for the other unpleasant surprise. Once the staff had wheeled me into the surgery room, I had to lift myself and climb from the gurney onto the operating table. I guess at 360 pounds, the skinny nurses weren't inclined to risk a hernia lifting and moving me. Although it was physically uncomfortable, especially given my size, weight, and sedated condition, the transition went well. Once my arms and legs were tied down securely, I allowed myself to relax, started to breathe deeply, and then my awareness faded away.

About two hours later, I awoke from surgery in the hospital's recovery room. My surgeon told me that the procedure had gone very well—a textbook case. I was transported on a gurney from the recovery area to my private room for my joyful, tearful reunion with Kari. We both thanked God for keeping me alive as I passed from the Gaining Side to the Losing Side.

Once installed in my wonderful hospital bed—capable of flexing and moving at the touch of a button in whatever direction was most helpful or comfortable—I wasn't feeling much pain from the incision and stapling (at least until I had to move). The most difficult challenges I faced during those first hours post-op were coping with the awful and constant discomfort of the nasal-gastric tube, pumping yucky stomach acids from my newly stapled stomach, and a terrible persistent dryness in my mouth. I wasn't permitted to drink or eat anything until the next day, after the doctors were assured that my stomach staples were holding fast and that there was no leakage out of my stomach.

Hospital staff soon came into my room and installed an ingenious trapeze contraption that turned out to be a real blessing and valuable tool. There were parallel bars above me; bracing bars on a slant; and a triangle bar in front that I could grasp and use to raise, lower, and shift out of bed, using my arm strength.

My doctor insisted that I start moving my body *immediately*. No rest for the weary! He required me to take a minimum of four walks around the ward in the first several hours after my surgery. Dr. Weber explained that this movement was vital, both to prevent dangerous embolisms and to get my stomach working again after the trauma of the stapling and surgery.

I was so grateful to have Kari's help in mastering the fine art of getting in and out of the bed to take my walks. It also proved to be invaluable to have Kari with me throughout that awful first day, attending to my needs, getting help when I needed it, and encouraging and assisting me to get out of bed and walk. We were soon able to figure out how best to use the trapeze apparatus to achieve this vital goal.

Kari would raise the head of the bed until I could grab the parallel bars; then I learned how to use my arms to pull and push myself up, and to shift my feet out and over the edge of bed and onto the floor. It was very slow going. Every time I got out of the bed to walk, we had to remove the intermittent compression pump attached to my lower legs to prevent embolisms; maneuver around the cords of the TV and the medical equipment in the room; bring along my IV drip for the trip; and move the furniture around to make a clear path into and out of the room. Somehow, it worked.

Initially I leaned on a wheelchair in front of me as I slowly circumnavigated the ward. With each step, and with each walk, I felt stronger and more confident. It also gave me something useful I could do, which was a valuable byproduct for a driven guy like me. I exceeded my four-walk goal that first day, and every day thereafter. I told myself that the pain multiplied my gain, and it worked.

Then, when I got back to my room after walking, I would sit down as far up and across the bed as possible, use the apparatus to simultaneously swing my legs up, and push off the foot of the bed, lifting myself by using the handles above while Kari pulled the mattress pad to reposition me in the center of the bed. Then she would lower the head of the bed while I held onto the triangle and lowered myself slowly back into position. I would then hit the blessed morphine button and collapse for a rest.

The respiratory therapist introduced me to the incentive barometer, a breathing apparatus whereby I worked constantly to maintain and increase the depth of my breathing. This turned out to be a really important tool: I was experiencing a low-grade fever, and the constant effort to expand my lung capacity helped me heal faster. I am convinced that my determination to meet and exceed each of my medical team's goals (for both walking and deep breathing) substantially expedited and promoted my rapid healing and recovery.

With the morphine drip, pain was *not* a problem. The discomfort of the gastric nasal tube and the extreme dryness of my mouth, however, were so severe that I found myself, several times, questioning whether the procedure had been worth it. That was probably a silly and irrational inquiry, but, as I've noted before, patience is not one of my strongest character assets. What got me through the initial ordeal was remembering the advice of a colleague who had preceded me in having the surgery. She reminded me that this extreme discomfort was a very time-limited phenomenon. I focused all my energies on getting through this phase.

I was very grateful that Kari sacrificed her comfort and sleep to spend the night cramped in the chair in my room. Her reassuring presence made all the difference in the world for me, and underscored the importance of having my own personal advocate and support system, especially for that first day and night.

During that first evening post-op, it seemed as if I was constantly being awoken, interrupted, monitored, treated, inspected, and assessed. Every staff member seemed to have their own specialized form of torture and disruption—measuring my blood pressure, checking my temperature, monitoring my IV drip, pricking me to check my blood sugars and insulin, checking my breathing, watching my oxygen levels, and so on.

One of my greatest challenges that first night post-op—and for many weeks thereafter—was sleeping without my CPAP machine. My doctor had insisted that I stop using the CPAP immediately after the operation because the force of the air pressure could conceivably disrupt my new stomach staples before they had a chance to settle in and stabilize. This was the first time in more than a decade that I slept (or tried to sleep) without my CPAP, and it was a scary task. I persisted in my irrational fear that if I fell asleep without the CPAP, I would die. It made sense to me at the time. Fortunately, Kari (the best planner in the world) had brought my radio, and between her soft voice, some cool jazz on the radio, and my ever-present new friend, the morphine drip, I made it through the night.

Yes, it hurt to move, walk, and even breathe, but once I got through the pain, I actually began to derive satisfaction from *doing everything in my power to make my WLS work*. Dr. Weber had promised me before the surgery that if I followed his instructions carefully and precisely, I would reach my goal weight and be a thin man within one year. I kept my eye on *the prize*.

Day Two

I awoke exhausted but thrilled to be alive. Having Kari at my side confirmed that this was not a dream, but a reality. I was fiercely determined to set new hospital records for second-day post-op walking and deep breathing capacity. However, there were other challenges still to be met and conquered before I could indulge my record-setting fantasies.

I was told that at 10:30 AM I would undergo an X-ray to check my stomach staples and make sure that there was no leakage. I would swallow a barium drink, which would leave a traceable trail through my stomach and digestive system, and the X-ray would confirm whether or not the staples were holding tight. Once I passed the test, the nurses would remove the very uncomfortable nasal-gastric tube, I could begin consuming beverages, and the rest of my recovery process would begin. This gave me something to aim for, and that "carrot" helped me get through the morning. Hunger was not my issue; instead, it was discomfort and impatience.

Unfortunately, several emergencies postponed the test until 2 PM, which seemed at the time to be a distant eternity. My faith in Dr. Weber and the very kind and responsive hospital staff helped me make it through. Once again, my limited patience was severely tested as I counted down the hours until the test could be completed and relief could be obtained.

I used the extra time to walk, walk, and walk some more, and to breathe so deeply that I would test the limits of the incentive barometer. The attendant brought me to the X-ray room in a wheelchair, where I encountered another challenge and momentary panic. In order to conduct the barium test, I had to stand for ten minutes, without anything to lean on, and then I had to shift my body in different directions to yield different perspectives on my stomach while they X-rayed the barium flow. I worried about the next challenge—climbing onto a step and from there onto a table for further examination. It was scary, but, again, my motivation overpowered my pain. Fortunately, the X-ray revealed that the surgery had been perfect, and that the staples were holding firm and steadfast.

The reward for moving through my pain and anxiety was the removal of the nasal-gastric tube. I won't linger on the details of the slimy, disgusting, stinky process, but before I knew it the tube had been removed. I was ever so grateful! Now I could blow my nose, suck on some ice chips, which tasted far better than any sugar treat had ever been, and sip a little water. Kari smeared Vaseline on my dry and parched lips and brushed my teeth and tongue, which felt as if they had been coated with yuck for weeks, not hours. The denta-swabs were great, and Kari kindly wiped my mouth and lips with a damp washcloth, which offered disproportionate delight after my first day's ordeal. This may not sound particularly appetizing, but in my condition, it was almost heaven!

The pace of my recovery really picked up speed on Day Two. Instead of focusing on the dual discomforts of my dry mouth and nasal-gastric tube, I was able to redirect my energies into my deep breathing exercises and walking excursions. I began to master the routine of using the overhead apparatus to swing out of my bed without assistance and, gathering my IV tower and other tubes and wires, walked around the ward until I knew every room, every floor tile, and every wall decoration intimately. I encountered Dr. Weber in the middle of a particularly impressive walk, and he was so pleased with my progress that he told me that I could choose to leave the hospital at the end of my third day (and second night) in the hospital.

This news cheered me immeasurably. I hate being in hospitals and yearned for the comforts (and privacy) of home. Also, the sooner I checked out of the hospital, the more money we could save in noncovered hospitalization costs.

By my second evening of "incarceration," Kari was so exhausted from her 24/7 care of me during my first two days in the hospital that she decided to spend the night in a real bed in a local motel. I encouraged and supported her in this decision, but I must admit I had some anxiety about being left on my own.

I need not have worried. I was able to get into and out of the bed without assistance; could do pretty much whatever I needed to do (including visits to the bathroom) on my own; and had developed trust in the staff to help with whatever I couldn't handle. Besides the pain-killing morphine, my intravenous drip provided me with hydration and nutrition, so I was urinating several times a day. The nurses and orderlies cheered as my body produced visible proof that I was progressing well.

Day Three

My recovery proceeded at an exponential rate. After I awoke on my third morning in the hospital, I was able to sit in a chair, instead of being confined to my bed. The smallest pleasures were disproportionately joyful! Later that morning, the nurses removed my IV. That meant that I would henceforth be responsible for feeding and hydrating myself. The good news: I was much more mobile without having to drag the IV tower on my walks. The bad news: this was the end of my morphine drip. It had been my dear friend and companion, but it was time to let go and move on.

When Dr. Weber arrived for his daily visit to monitor my condition, he set the terms and conditions for my recovery after leaving the hospital that evening. He wanted me to walk, at a comfortable pace, at least one hour a day, every day, and to increase both pace and distance as best I could. He prescribed a protein-laden drink for the next few days, as well as pain medications to pick up where the morphine drip left off. He instructed me to consume one ounce of food (clear liquids or pureed concoctions) every thirty minutes for the next several days, and advised me to add dairy, citrus, and warm liquid beverages thereafter. We set our first post-op appointment for two weeks after my release from the hospital. Although I could shower, he cautioned against changing the bandage over my wounds. Finally, he prescribed a significantly lower dose of insulin than I had been taking before my surgery, and encouraged me to check my blood sugars frequently.

I achieved my desired early release from the hospital by 9:30 PM on my third day in the hospital (about sixty hours after my admission) so that we could minimize our hospital bills.

I weighed 336 pounds when I left the hospital (down twenty-four pounds in my first three days of post-op)!

While I cursed my health plan's shortsighted and counterproductive refusal to pay for the procedure that necessitated my rush to check out, I remained grateful for the opportunity to reduce our out-of-pocket costs. We returned to Kari's motel room for the night. My pain and discomfort were excruciating—trying to sleep on a flat bed after what I now appreciated as the blessing of an adjustable hospital bed—but I made it (barely) through the night. At 4 AM I could bear it no longer, and Kari was rested enough to safely drive the three hours back to our home.

Kari's Advice to In-Hospital Caregivers and Advocates

When I subsequently asked Kari for her suggestions for spouses, partners, family members, or friends acting as in-hospital caregivers and advocates helping their loved ones through the weight loss surgery process, she offered the following recommendations, which may prove useful.

- It's important for caregivers to be assertive, but not pushy, with the medical team on the ward. The staff is so busy that they must prioritize care, thereby postponing attention to a patient with lesser needs, wants, or discomforts. The caregiver can provide the gentle prods and reminders that will expedite attention. Respectfully asking for what you want and need will almost always produce better results than not asking.

- "Do for the patient" at the very beginning of their post-op recovery in the hospital, but always look for ways to encourage and empower them to do for themselves. The sooner and the more independent the WLS patient becomes, the more their recovery will be expedited.

- Watch and learn from the nurses. While, of course, they remain responsible for monitoring and using the medical apparatuses, tasks like removing the patient's leg airbags, unraveling and straightening out the IV cords, and helping the patient get out of bed and take a walk can then be done without the nurse's help, thereby allowing patients to do more when they feel like doing it, rather than having to wait for assistance.

• It is vital for the caregiver, if at all possible, to spend at least the first day, the first night, and even next day as the patient's 24/7 observer, helper, and advocate. At the same time, it may prove helpful for the (by then) exhausted caregiver to get a good night's sleep away from the hospital on the second and subsequent nights of hospitalization. This encourages (and forces) the patient to begin functioning more independently (e.g., getting out of bed, going to the bathroom, and walking the ward on their own.)

My First Weeks and Months of Post-Op Recovery at Home

Even on the drive home, and in my first days back at home, many of my new post-op challenges quickly emerged.

I received and enjoyed brief phone calls from family and friends checking on my recovery. They needed reassurance that I was going to be alright, and I was pleased to be able to give them the comfort they sought. I soon became frustrated, however, with the disparity between sounding so good and strong on the phone, even as I continued the deep, dark questioning of my choice and my prospects.

My wound pain turned out to be one of the least of my problems. The prescribed pain medications helped greatly, and I found that as long as I continued to walk at least sixty minutes each day (the distance and speed increasing progressively as I moved further away from my surgery), the pain from the incisions and stapling was relatively easy to manage. The more I walked, the less I hurt. I often used the incentive barometer to improve and maintain my lung functioning, and this too seemed to significantly ease my pain and expedite my healing. I can honestly report that within seven to ten days of my return home, the pain was receding and stopped being a major concern.

Other post-op consequences were much harder for me. Of course, every body is different, and reacts and heals differently. Lots of my fellow WLS-ers reported having a much faster and easier recovery than I experienced. Reports from colleagues who chose the increasingly popular and minimally intrusive laparoscopic forms of weight loss surgery suggested dramatically shorter and easier recoveries.

For me, however, the post-op problems I experienced in those first days and weeks were sufficiently severe and disturbing to keep me questioning whether I had made the right choice in having the surgery. I have a fairly high pain threshold and tolerance, but several aspects of my recovery were devastatingly debilitating.

For example, I was constantly nauseous. Nothing (including a powerful anti-nausea drug used by chemotherapy patients) seemed to help, other than time. My sense of smell seemed somehow heightened after my surgery, and virtually anything that Kari cooked increased my nausea. Even watching the endless parade of TV advertisements for food and restaurants turned my stomach. I never realized how completely saturated TV was with ads pushing sugar and refined junk foods.

A week after my surgery, I was still seriously questioning whether I had made a colossal mistake. The constant nausea, diarrhea, and sleep deprivation were taking their toll on my body and my spirits. On top of that, the weight was not exactly pouring off. It felt like more of a trickle.

I suffered from extreme sleep deprivation, and without question that prolonged my discomfort and delayed my full recovery and return to work. After sleeping with a CPAP for more than a decade, I found it difficult, if not impossible, to sleep without the machine. Part of my difficulty was psychological; I had become so psychologically dependent on the CPAP to keep my air passages open and ensure that my breathing continued without interruption that I was terrified of falling asleep, even as my body cried out for rest.

It was also quite a formidable challenge to find any comfortable position or way to sleep. Much of that time is still a blurry haze in my memory, but I recall what seemed to be endless nights propped up in my recliner or on the living room sofa with pillows and cushions, tossing and turning and trying to find a position that didn't hurt and would allow me to sleep. I drifted in and out of sleep amid the endless racket of satellite TV movies and news shows. I moved from sofa to chair and back again, seriously questioning whether I would *ever* sleep normally again.

Of course, I did. A breakthrough came, about two weeks post-op, when another WLS patient I was corresponding with, and who had experienced similar problems sleeping, suggested a sleeping pill that had worked well for him. After consulting with my bariatric surgeon, and gaining his approval, I obtained a prescription from my family doctor, and soon I was sleeping through the night, once again, in my own bed. What a blessed relief! I was just sorry that I had suffered for so long before reaching out and asking more experienced WLS veterans for help. I learned from that mistake!

I followed my surgeon's directions precisely with respect to the timing and sequence of each step up the "food chain" ladder. My first major food crisis happened about two weeks after surgery, when his nutrition guidelines suggested that

I was ready to try scrambled eggs. That was the first (but most definitely not the last) time that I learned, from very painful experience, that eating too fast, or too much, or eating foods that, for whatever reason, my testy tummy couldn't handle, would result in an indescribable combination of upset stomach, nausea, unbearable fullness, and discomfort.

Nothing would relieve my discomfort until I forced myself to vomit up the eggs I couldn't tolerate. While it's not a pleasant experience, it's proved to be the *only* way I've been able to obtain relief (within an hour or so) from the unbearable agony of being blocked up or backed up, at least when walking fails to resolve the agony.

There were other problems that plagued my first weeks of recovery. I experienced constant and exhausting bouts of diarrhea. I lagged behind schedule in making the planned and expected transition from clear liquids to liquids to soft foods to real foods. As my recovery lagged, and as I continued to be so sick and tired, I was having a real problem consuming enough water. My stomach simply didn't seem willing or able to accommodate the 120 ounces of water my doctor wanted me to drink daily. I couldn't gulp; I could only sip. And even constant sipping didn't seem to adequately hydrate my body. Accordingly, I suffered from…constipation!

I was also surprised to find myself feeling very depressed. Depression had *not* been a major issue for me before the surgery, and I worried that my depression might become yet another long-term problem. I learned, again through the invaluable network of WLS e-mail groups and forums, that it's quite common for WLS patients to experience depression, especially when they're still suffering in the initial recovery period dominated by pain, diarrhea, sleep deprivation, nausea, and the other normal manifestations of healing from surgical trauma.

Finally, I had lots of problems adjusting my insulin dosages to suit my new body and its changing needs. Initially, I was taking too much insulin (even at the reduced levels my doctor suggested), and I paid a price—that nightmare of a "crash." My blood sugars were too low, and that left me feeling weak and sick. Then I overreacted and took too little insulin, and my blood sugar levels were unacceptably high.

Two weeks after my surgery, I was relieved to meet with Dr. Weber. The primary purpose of the appointment was for him to remove the external staples binding together my surgery incision, running from below my breastbone and extending down my stomach. The wound was healing well, and although the removal of the staples burned a bit, the process was quick and relatively painless. My secondary purpose was to get a reality check: was recovery so difficult for all, most, or many patients? My doctor reassured me that I was healing well; doing all the right things; and the nausea would soon begin to recede. (It did.) I was thrilled to learn that I had now lost thirty pounds in my first two weeks post-op.

The good news and the validation of both my suffering and the likelihood that it would start dramatically improving soon, cheered me immeasurably. My pain and discomfort became much easier to handle and accept now that I knew that I would feel much better soon. I was also pleased that he told me I could now resume my water walking and aerobics to supplement my daily walking, and that I could once again join Kari for our magical time together in our hot tub, set under the stars and gazing directly up into the snow-covered peaks of the Olympic Mountain Range.

Just as Dr. Weber predicted, I started feeling dramatically better soon after the two-week anniversary of my surgery. I finally felt that I had turned the corner, and that my recovery would be much easier, smoother, and more productive from this point on. I started feeling noticeably better each and every day. My nausea disappeared; my increasingly vigorous daily exercise was improving my metabolic burn; and I was on target for consistently losing twenty pounds or more each month.

As if by magic, one month to the day after my surgery, my recovery and progress started improving at an exponential rate. My daily and long-term blood sugar scores were approaching normal levels. Kari and I resumed (carefully at first) playing, traveling, going to movies, and doing "normal" things. I was, at long last, laughing, playing, and starting to feel like a human being again. I still had to pace myself, and carefully monitor both my food intake and my activities to avoid extreme discomfort or fatigue. But my life was finally returning to normal. The weight was now pouring off. My pre-op clothes no longer fit. I moved down one size and celebrated by completing my longest walk to date (two miles).

From that day on, vigorous walking became part of my daily routine. And as my excess weight continued to disappear, the pain that had always been associated with walking melted away. Walking became something that was both fun and one of the best things I could do to feel good and to expedite my weight loss.

I have a type-A, or driven, personality and am a lifelong workaholic. Before my surgery, and based on the accounts of other patients and the observations of my bariatric surgeon, I expected to be up and running and back to work full time within two to four weeks of my surgery. I decided that for a man with my heretofore legendary drive and stamina, two weeks would be more than enough recovery time. It wasn't.

It was a full eight weeks before I felt strong and well enough to start working part-time, and it was ten weeks post-op before I felt like myself. Again, every *body* is different. I've subsequently talked to many WLS-ers (especially those who had the less intrusive laparoscopic procedures) who were back at work, full-steam ahead, in one or two weeks. And I've encountered many folks who needed a much longer recovery time. It's important to avoid comparisons, and to know that a body will take whatever time it needs to recover. This is something that can't be rushed.

Again, trust, faith, and patience were all character assets that were as limited, in my case, as my girth was huge. It was, to put it mildly, a valuable learning experience for me.

Whatever I lacked in trust, faith, and patience, however, I was blessed with in love, nurturance, reassurance, and the help of my wife and partner, Kari. For those terrible first several weeks of recovery, I relied totally on her to prepare my meals and the protein drinks that proved to be my salvation, to juggle my medications and vitamins, and to otherwise nurse me through my personal hell of healing. Kari paid a terrible price for her unstinting caregiving. She has suffered for fifteen years from chronic fatigue syndrome, and yet she summoned the strength and stamina to get me through. It took her months to recover from this caregiving—far longer than it took me to once again fully feel like myself.

I couldn't have made it through without her. It was her unstinting love and support that made it possible for me to heal, recover, and move ahead with the ultimate task that lay ahead—losing the rest of my excess weight and keeping it off.

3

My Transformation

Through Thick and Thin #8
(After the Surgery—3 weeks)

My First View from the Losing Side
or
I'm Glad I've Made It Here, But It Was a Very Bumpy Ride

Today is the first day that I have felt enough strength, energy, clarity, and focus to share my perspective about this transformative journey. My bottom line: I'm glad I had the surgery *and* this trip has been far more painful, agonizing, and difficult than I ever imagined it would be. I seemed to have invested most of my energy in preparing for the surgery, without ever understanding how nasty a ride these first few weeks would be. I'm starting to believe the prediction I've heard: I will need a full week of recovery for each of the four days I was required to be in the hospital.

Here are three important things I've learned about myself that I want to share before I collapse back into my recliner and resume dreaming and scheming about easing back into work next week.

- The scale is my enemy, not my friend, and will sabotage me if I let it. I don't have my own scale (I threw it out many years ago when I first realized that compulsive dieting and weighing were part of my weight problem). So the first time that I weighed myself after surgery was at my ten-day checkup with my doctor. I was thrilled to note a thirty-pound weight loss in those ten days. And I was so proud of myself for waiting another whole week before stopping at my doctor's office for another weigh-in. When the scale showed *zero* additional weight loss, I immediately spun off into panic and despair. Why had I gone through this hell if it wasn't going to work for me? Of course, Kari, my angel, asked all the right questions. How often was I having bowel movements? Once I realized that I had been constipated for a week, I was able to figure out that the combined effects of the anesthesia and my liquid pain medications were plugging me tighter than my belt used to fit around my waistline. So I've done all the right things—stopped or switched my medications, started taking daily doses of prune juice and mineral oil, sipped a different tea, increased my water consumption and hydration, and so on. Now I'm once again releasing my lost weight through bowel movements and physical movement of my body. I began to see the first trap I had fallen into—measuring my success by the number registering on the scale. I will no longer be held hostage to the terrorism of the scale or judge the validity of my WLS decision by counting, in the short term, how many pounds I've lost.

- Each person is absolutely unique and different. Post-op experiences and consequences will differ. Recovery and recuperative periods will differ. Weight and inches are lost at different speeds. I will not compare my weight loss, by total poundage, rate of loss, or other such formulas, to those of others. That is surely the path to insanity and self-sabotage for me.

- While I work toward my goal of healthful longevity, comfort, and happiness, I will speak my truth about WLS to those who want to know of my experience. And, in the process, I will make special efforts to fully disclose and describe all aspects—both good and bad.

I can feel myself coming back. I'm starting to have thoughts about resuming work. I'm planning to surprise Kari with an excursion to the movies tomorrow. I'm accepting more phone calls than I'm refusing. And this is still one of the most physically, emotionally, and spiritually difficult challenges I've ever undertaken. I'm glad I did it, but I'm even more glad to be moving out of the valleys and starting to trek toward the peaks.

Through Thick and Thin #9
(After the Surgery—1 Month)

My Gratitude Attitude at Thanksgiving

Thanksgiving is one of my favorite holidays because it gives me an annual opportunity to count my blessings, and to recultivate the *gratitude attitude* that I strive to carry throughout my daily life. Here's what I'm most grateful for this Thanksgiving:

- I'm grateful that I survived my surgery, that I'm healing well, and that I'm well on my way to healthful fitness. The scale tells me I've lost more than forty pounds (11% of my pre-op weight) in this first month. The tape documents that I've lost more than two feet worth of inches around my neck, chest, waist, thighs, and ankles. I can feel my body reshaping and transforming. I'm enjoying a vigorous 1.5-mile walk every day. I don't think much about food, and sometimes I even forget to eat. I'm grateful for all these things—and for the medical folks who worked so skillfully to help me harvest these miracles.

- I'm grateful that I have a partner, Kari, who has nursed me—in every sense of that word—through a very difficult first month of recovery. In some ways, I'm a model patient: doing my daily exercise, sticking to the prescribed liquid food plan, etc. In most other ways, however, I'm a stubborn, negative, pessimistic, depressive, helpless, hopeless, and impatient patient. Kari has been the one who has comforted and cared, nurtured and nourished, listened and laughed, cheered and cajoled, and otherwise done whatever was required to get me to listen to my body when it's been telling me that it's not yet ready to return to work. I have fought her, every day for one month, wanting to work and perform responsibilities that my body has not yet been ready to undertake. I'm so grateful that Kari understands me better than I understand myself, and that she's somehow been able to penetrate my maze of rationalizations, denials, pretenses, and ignorance so that I've taken the time (albeit kicking and screaming) that I've needed to heal and restore.

- I'm grateful for the inexpressible joy I experienced, two nights ago, when we went through my entire wardrobe and donated 95% of it to our local charity thrift shop. It was not just the joy of seeing, feeling, and believing that my clothes were too big for me, but it was also the joy of trying on those gorgeous shirts, pants, sweaters, jackets, and suits that I had optimistically boxed up and stored over the years in my insane hope that maybe someday I would lose the weight. What a sublime feeling to feel the formerly unfitting clothes hug and caress my body as if they had been hand-tailored! How handsome and trim, how attractive and thin I felt as I modeled my "new" recycled wardrobe and hung it proudly in my closet. And I'm grateful, in advance, for the day when these clothes will hang from me and I'll need to buy new clothes, off the rack.

- I'm grateful for the community of WLS-ers who have been there for me, every step of the way, to inform, encourage, and support me on my path from morbid obesity to healthful fitness. I'm grateful too for all the people who are still considering the surgery or those who are beginners like me—they give me a reason to keep on writing and sharing my experiences, dips, strength, and hope.

- I'm grateful to my God and to the Universe for giving me this second chance to transform my body and thereby my health, fitness, comfort, and living experience. I'm grateful for all the spiritual, emotional, and practical help I've gotten that has enabled me to really, truly get it, that using WLS to resolve my morbid obesity problem is a logical, reasonable, and entirely appropriate strategy, utilizing an increasingly safe and effective medical procedure. And that this is most certainly not taking the easy way out, not a source of embarrassment or shame, and not a badge or symptom of weakness or failure.

- Last, but not least, I'm grateful for my courage, and for my ability to listen to and trust my still small voice within that has moved me down this path.

Through Thick and Thin #10
(After the Surgery—2 Months)

The View from Eight Weeks Out
or
I'm So Surprised I'm Still Fat When I Look in the Mirror

How completely different, and how wonderful, things look today! The pain, frustrations, and challenges of my difficult first six weeks of recuperation have already begun to recede, and I'm feeling better, stronger, thinner, and more myself each day.

I have now lost more than fifty pounds and, when I weigh myself, I expect to weigh less than 300 pounds for the first time in many decades. My diabetes has virtually disappeared (i.e., my blood sugar counts four times a day are invariably normal). My severe case of obstructive sleep apnea (which had kept me chained at night to my CPAP for more than a decade) is also close to disappearing as a result of my weight loss.

Each of these changes is a blessing and a miracle. Another wonder is the fact that I am vigorously walking at least two miles each day and loving it! I feel more fit with every step. Every week I increase my pace and speed, and I hope to be able to comfortably walk five miles by my six-month anniversary. My next unimaginable goal is to be able to complete a very difficult ten-mile hike through a pristine old-growth forest by next summer.

I am just beginning my transition from a purely liquid diet to solid foods. It's been difficult for me to slow the pace of my eating. But I've been blessed by a lack of hunger pangs between meals. I still struggle to tolerate any variety of solid and semisolid foods. (I've been surprised, yet I feel validated to learn that many others also experience such severe limitations in their food options.) I've turned the need to chew my food into a liquid state into an exercise in sensuous eating, savoring every last drop—and that's working!

The greatest miracle of all has been having and feeling an operational appetite regulator.

I can now recognize the feeling that tells me when I'm full. When I experience that feeling, I stop eating immediately to avoid the unpleasant sensations of feeling stuffed. I've yearned for a working appetite regulator my whole life, and I feel so fortunate today to have one that's really working for me. And I'm proud and pleased that I'm developing a new habit of stopping my eating as soon as I feel the "full" message.

What a joy it is to feel my body morphing, reshaping, and transforming, to have already baggy clothes become even baggier, and to know that absolutely everything in my wardrobe fits me splendidly, or loosely, and that I'll soon be ready for the next tier of sizes.

The strangest experience I've had, amid all these miracles, is the shock and disbelief I experience when I happen to catch a glimpse of myself in the mirror. I feel like I'm already at my goal weight of 180, moving with grace and style, but then I'm confronted with this image of a still very obese man in the mirror. It just doesn't compute. And I know that it's just a matter of time until the two images merge together and the thin man I feel like shows up in my thin image in the mirror.

Through Thick and Thin #11
(After the Surgery—3 Months)

The End of My Love Affair with Food

I'm continuing to work my program with commitment and intensity, and my program is continuing to work for me. I've lost almost seventy pounds (almost 20 percent of my highest weight). My sleep apnea is gone. My diabetes is controlled through diet and exercise, not insulin. When Kari and I hug, our bodies are close and form an "H," not an "A." And I'm starting now to consistently receive and savor the compliments of friends and associates who appreciate the difference in my face, body, and wardrobe.

There's just one thing I find myself missing and grieving: the end of my life-long love affair with the drama, smell, taste, texture, appearance, and excitement of food. My eating program, which is working well for me, is pretty boring and bland: yogurt for breakfast; tea throughout the morning, and my soy protein milkshakes (flavored with frozen berries) for lunch and mid-afternoon snack deliver an awesome sixty grams of very low-calorie protein. And then one to three teeny, tiny, innocuous ounces of solid food for dinner—divided into nine smaller piles and eaten five minutes per pile. Perhaps my dinner consists of an ounce or more of salmon (high in beneficial omega-3) or free-range chicken mixed with mayonnaise, some slivers of veggies, and some slices of fruit. If I need a mid-evening snack, I enjoy sherbet, half of a graham cracker. or a fig Newton.

Now, let me be clear: *I'm not complaining.* I am positively joyful with the exchange I've made: weight loss, increased mobility, decreased body pain, and improved appearance vs. cheap thrills. I'm just noticing how much I have been mourning the loss of the sizzle (mostly mental) of "real food." Sometimes I catch myself starting to sit on the pity pot of "I'll never be able to eat a super-giant cheeseburger or deli sandwich with the works" again.

A small bit of consolation: I find that I can still remember clearly the delicious aroma and taste of many of those foods that used to thrill me—like a great steak, pastrami sandwich, BBQ, corn on the cob, and French fries—and I can *almost* derive satisfaction from simply *savoring the memory* of their consumption.

I notice my food grief especially during social meals in restaurants. I've found some great coping mechanisms (like ordering a cup of soup and taking such tiny sips that I can stretch it out for the thirty to forty minutes it takes everyone else to complete their multicourse meal). I never realized how much of a role food plays in these elaborate social rituals and interactions called "going out for dinner."

Recently I was on the road for a week on business. I was amazed at how simple my life had become with the elimination of the infinite variety of food choices. I'm also gratified by how much money I save by drinking tap water and walking instead of eating.

The important thing is that this grief and mourning will soon pass, whereas my weight loss and improved fitness promise a prolonged lifetime of joy and health. I can live without this particular love affair. And that's why I'm loving myself more each day as I carefully eat and exercise my way to fitness and longevity.

Through Thick and Thin #12
(After the Surgery—3.5 Months)

Why I'm Succeeding with Weight Loss Surgery When Nothing Else Worked

1. I now have a well-functioning appetite regulator.

Before my surgery, my appetite was voracious and without limit. I'm not sure how and when my natural, built-in appetite regulator stopped functioning (or maybe it never did work right), but my appetite for food was a hole that was literally never filled. I never ate to the point where I was so full that I vomited, but I was always able to stretch my stomach to accommodate my insatiable appetite for food. When I stopped eating, it was because my mind made a judgment that enough was enough, and I consciously acted as if I felt full, even though I didn't.

Today, and ever since my surgery, my appetite regulator works exceedingly well. I've discovered that my body needs surprisingly little food to fuel my activities and keep me well. I feel real hunger pangs when my stomach is empty, and I need food to maintain or raise my healthy blood sugar levels. I've learned that I can trust those cues—unlike the pangs of emotional hunger that I used to feel incessantly. I've learned to recognize what a full stomach feels like and, through behavioral conditioning, I've learned to stop eating instantly when I feel full.

2. Behavioral conditioning works for me.

Like a dog in one of Pavlov's experiments, I've become conditioned by adverse consequences to avoid overeating. A very small amount of food fills me to the point where even one more bite would make my stomach feel queasy, stuffed, and uncomfortable—and possibly prompt vomiting. This is a very unpleasant sensation. Also, vomiting adversely affects my physical state of being for hours afterward, so I have learned to do whatever it takes to avoid it. This means I stop eating instantly, or else pay the painful and unacceptable price.

3. Positive feedback works for me.

Every day when I feel my incredible shrinking body, when I see my weight decline on the once-dreaded scale, when clothes fit my diminishing dimensions, when I receive compliments and encouragement from others, when I can walk faster and farther than ever before, when I feel like a thin man—all this positive feedback encourages me to divert my energy from obsessing about or craving food. Instead, I bask in the satisfaction of finally, after all these years and all these unfulfilled commitments, moving toward my goal of health and fitness. Interestingly, I don't often feel deprived or denied about the current, severe constraints on my eating. Instead, I've made a conscious intellectual and emotional commitment to relegate food to a very minor role in my personal hierarchy of pleasure sources.

On the one hand, there's my relatively sparse, bland, and boring food plan. On the other hand, I'm achieving so many of my personal goals—becoming healthy and fit, eliminating my comorbid conditions, living without so much pain, and prolonging my life. The contest isn't even close.

Other veterans of WLS advise me that my stomach pouch will expand, that there will come a time when I can eat enough, and with glorious variety, to restore some of the emotional excitement formerly associated with food. But honestly, for me and for today, I am very happy to be bored with my food and thrilled with my life.

Through Thick and Thin #13
(After the Surgery—3.75 Months)

WLS Peaks and Plateaus

I don't need any help dealing with my WLS peaks—dramatic weight loss; improving health and fitness; freedom from blood sugar pricks, insulin, and the CPAP; shrinking circumferences; compliments; and praise. These are a few of my favorite things, and they are very easy to handle. However, dealing with my present weight plateau is a real challenge.

Over these last few weeks (midway through my fourth month post-op), I have experienced a sudden and disturbing plateau in my weight loss. The scale tells me I haven't lost a pound in two weeks, after sustained periods during which I averaged losing one pound a day. Nothing about my weight loss and fitness program has changed, except for the results. I'm continuing to vigorously walk 1.5–3.5 miles daily, and I'm eating healthy foods in very small and prudent amounts.

Maintaining faith, trust, and a positive attitude are my challenges when the scale doesn't move. The first place I tend to go is toward guilt and shame. It's like that's my default setting. I must be doing something wrong. I guess so many years of assaulting myself with blame about my morbid obesity have created a reflexive reaction. Yet I know, on a rational level, there's no basis for guilt. I'm doing everything right; I'm being careful with my caloric intake and consistent with my caloric burns from exercise.

When I reject my initial feelings of guilt, blame, and shame, I seem to turn next to skepticism and cynicism. I must be the sole exception to the rule. WLS surgery won't work for me. It's all over. Despair. Helpless and hopeless.

And then I listen to my still small inner voice. I listen to my wife. I listen to what my peers are sharing in the e-mail groups. I reread the WLS books, and my bible—*The Long-Term Success Habits of Gastric Bypass Patients*. I call my doctor's office for reassurance. I recalculate my caloric intake to make sure that it's appropriately low. I redouble my efforts to hydrate my body with water. I repeat my affirmation mantras with increased fervor. I redouble my commitment to exercise. And then, slowly, I begin to regain my confidence, hope, and optimism.

Apparently most people experience periodic plateaus after their WLS. My metabolism may be consolidating and shifting. It's also possible that my exercise is turning body fat into heavier solid muscle (that's how it feels and looks) and that might limit weight loss even as my body continues to grow slimmer and more fit.

Here are the two most important things I've decided to do to respond to this plateau: *to work on bolstering my faith and to stay away from the scale*. The latter may seem counterintuitive, since the scale may offer the only scientific, objective way to prove my continuing weight loss. But this strategy represents *my* path to serenity, sanity, and renewed trust. Focusing on the scale and the numbers feed my obsessive, compulsive, insanity-producing fears and anxieties. My addiction is to dieting. For me, for today, I'd rather trust than lust for the scale's reassurance.

I'll drop by my doctor's office when it's convenient, sometime in the next week or so, but until then I'll just keep working my program and strengthening my faith that my tiny tummy, my reduced caloric intake, and my enhanced caloric burns—a little less in, a little more out—will, in the long run, produce the 180-pound weight loss I seek.

Through Thick and Thin #14
(After the Surgery—4.25 Months)

Blocked!

It was a very scary and uncomfortable episode when my stomach became blocked. With help from my doctor's staff, I was finally able to dissolve the blockage by nightfall, by which time I was exhausted, famished, remorseful, and grateful. I learned a few useful strategies.

My problem started near bedtime one day as I was trying out a new brand of a chewable calcium supplement. I had run out of my favorite brand, which, besides being a convenient source of calcium, worked well to neutralize the bitter taste I experience when I crush my large prescribed pills and mix the powder with mineral oil to ease their way down.

Anyway, because I had to wait for a replacement package, I bought a different brand to use in the meantime. But I should have known better than to swallow it when I found it to be hard, not soft. I had to chew it forcefully to get it down. Soon thereafter I had the warning signs of upset stomach—nausea and imminent vomiting. The worst of the wave of discomfort passed and I went to bed, although the discomfort continued and I felt on the verge of vomiting for a few hours until I finally fell asleep.

The next morning, I should have paid closer attention: I should have remembered and linked the previous night's discomfort. However, when I awoke in the morning and downed my medication and mineral oil cocktail, I grabbed yet another tablet of the new supplement and chewed it nearly to death. Later that day, when Kari and I went to an Italian restaurant for lunch after a shopping excursion, I compounded my mistake. I ordered what seemed to be the most healthful soup on the menu, without registering that it contained bits of sausage. I had only a few slurps, and one well-chewed piece of sausage, before my stomach sent me unmistakable warning that it was very unhappy with my choices.

Soon I vomited up the soup, and for the rest of the afternoon and this second evening, I couldn't keep down either liquids or solid food. And my discomfort grew ominously to the point where I called my doctor's advice nurse for help. I was terrified that it was going to require a surgical intervention to remove the blockage.

The nurse explained that the combination of a heavier, denser calcium supplement and the fatty sausage were probably resisting digestion and blocking the exit from my stomach. She suggested that I limit my intake to more mineral oil—to lubricate the remaining contents of my stomach in order to ease its evacuation. She also suggested walking, so that gravity would help the elimination process. I did as I was told, although I felt so bad that walking even a short distance was a trial.

Within a few hours, the blockage was eliminated, the food moved on into my intestines, and I was able to sip some chicken soup broth to ease my hunger.

Throughout this episode, I continued to beat myself up for not paying attention, and for failing to learn from my mistakes:

- For failing to conduct an immediate investigation and analysis after I had trouble with the first chewable

- For failing to discard the supplements after my first difficult episode

- For failing to notice that the soup had sausage

- For failing to dish the sausage out of the soup and discard it

I am so quick to abuse myself when my learning curve is slow or impaired.

What I have learned (or more precisely re-learned) from my first blockage is the vital necessity of my staying aware, conscious, and vigilant about *absolutely everything* that I put in my mouth, and to stop immediately and figure out what's wrong at the very first signs of any problem. Just as I have learned to stop eating—*immediately*—when I feel full, and to avoid water during meals, and to avoid raw vegetables and fatty foods, I have now learned that if I fail to pay attention to my body's early warning system, I do so at my own peril.

I have also remembered that blame and shame serve absolutely no useful purpose and have no positive effect. I've resolved to try to take the energy I've used in blaming and shaming myself when I err and to reinvest that energy in staying aware, conscious, and vigilant.

Through Thick and Thin #15
(After the Surgery—4.75 Months)

The Agony and the Ecstasy

The irony would have been both exquisite and laughable if I didn't hurt so much. Last Tuesday evening, even as I shared with several newcomers to our WLS support group the reasons why I'm so grateful that I had this surgery, my nausea conspired with my hunger pangs to shorten my sharing. I felt terrible. I hadn't been able to keep anything down except for water and broth in the preceding seventy-two hours, and I was starting to experience the light-headed and weakened altered state I remembered from previous (voluntary) food fasts. And the situation got much worse before it got very much better.

Here's the story of my agony and ecstasy. It had been almost five months since my VBG and my very limited, bland, and boring eating plan was serving me well. I was rapidly approaching my 100-pound weight loss milestone, and feeling so good otherwise, that I wasn't particularly disturbed or bothered by the fact that my food choices remained severely circumscribed by my tiny and sensitive new tummy.

I wasn't unduly concerned last Saturday when my second post-op attempt to enjoy a small portion of eggs scrambled with cheese started me on a painful cycle of vomiting that was to continue for five days. On Sunday, I tried the mineral oil and walking. By Monday morning, I was on the phone with my doctor's office nurse again, starting to feel a bit desperate. I didn't have a fever so I knew it wasn't the flu or an infection. She suggested that I start from scratch again by drinking clear liquids and give it another day or two. By Thursday I was scared. With no change, I was still unable to keep food down, and my stomach was in spasm from all the upheavals. I was able to get an appointment with a doctor three hours away in Seattle (a recommendation from my VBG doctor, who was out of town) for a consult and, if necessary, a scoping of my esophagus, stomach pouch, and stoma. I wavered between believing that there was no problem (I was making this all up), and believing that I must have done something terribly wrong (I was always quick to blame myself).

After my Thursday morning consult, the doctor decided that something was wrong and scheduled the endoscopy for late afternoon. When I weighed myself at the hospital, I found that I had lost ten pounds during my ordeal, bringing me within three pounds of my 100-pound weight loss. By this time, however, I was feeling too much pain and fear to celebrate. This was *not* the way I wanted to lose my weight.

After giving me a potent gargle to numb my throat before they dropped the wire containing a camera down my esophagus and into my stomach pouch, the doctor gave me an anesthetic like the one I had during my last colonoscopy, and the next thing I knew the nurse was wheeling me into the recovery room where Kari and I met with the doctor. The news was initially chilling, and then thrilling.

It turns out that I have been experiencing a fairly severe case of acid reflux since my surgery, and that the excess of acidic digestive juices had caused ulcers within the lining of my reduced stomach pouch. A daily medication would heal the ulcers and prevent their future development. The acid reflux had apparently also complicated my efforts to eat and keep down a variety of other foods, and the doctor offered me hope that, once healed, I might be able to diversify my eating plan and enjoy some of the gastric delights I had consigned to the "can't eat" category.

That's the story of my agony and my ecstasy. The *pain and discomfort* amounted to an expensive price that fades from my memory quickly. The *hope* that I won't have to continue forever to be so stoic about my food options: priceless.

Through Thick and Thin #16
(After the Surgery—5 Months)

The Tale of the Tape Measure
or
The Numbers Speak for Themselves

To commemorate the date of my WLS, every month Kari and I enjoy our own special WLS post-op ritual: to carefully measure the changed circumferences of twelve different parts of my body. Five months after surgery, and having lost more than 100 pounds, here's the tale told by the tape. I'm happy to let the numbers speak for themselves:

- My head: −1 inch

- My neck: −4.5 inches

- My upper arm: −6.5 inches

- My lower arm: −1.5 inches

- My upper chest: −4 inches

- My chest, below my breasts: −8 inches

- My waist: −13.5 inches

- My hips: −9.5 inches

- My upper thighs: −6.25 inches

- My calves: −1.25 inches

- Above my knee: −3 inches

- My ankles: −1.5 inches

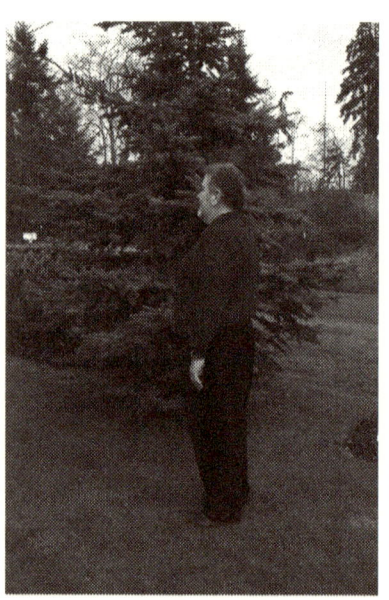

Total inches lost to date: 59.5 inches (five feet)

For most of my life, getting measured ranked right up there with getting weighed and shopping for extra-sized clothes. It's wonderful to see how WLS has transformed them all into treasured and joyful rituals!

Through Thick and Thin #17
(After the Surgery—6.25 Months)

The Top Ten Reasons Why Weight Loss Surgery is *Not* the "Easy Way Out"

10. It's very expensive. Many health insurance companies don't pay for the surgery, and even when they do, copayments and other costs add up quickly. Also, it can become very costly to constantly replenish wardrobes as the weight comes off.

9. Recovery can be very painful. Besides the pain from the surgery wound, patients may experience nausea or severe gastric distress. Patients with sleep apnea may become sleep deprived, with all the associated adverse affects, when they must discontinue use of their CPAP machines to avoid disturbing the staples creating their tiny new stomach pouch.

8. Recuperation can take a long time. Patients may be out of commission and absent from work for a prolonged period of recovery time. In some cases, patients may not be able to return to work or normal pursuits for up to ten or twelve weeks.

7. It's hard work and a major time commitment. For optimal results, patients should engage in aerobic exercise for one hour per day. For bodies unaccustomed to vigorous exercise, this can be very hard. It's also a real challenge for WLS patients to learn all they must about nutrition so they can ensure that their food and vitamins are sustaining their body. Finally, it can be exhausting to consciously, carefully, and painstakingly chew every bit of food that enters your mouth.

6. Vomiting isn't fun, nor is diarrhea. It may take patients many months (and frequent episodes of vomiting or diarrhea) to identify incompatible foods and to learn the practical limits of their newly reduced stomachs or digestive systems.

5. It takes extraordinary courage to consciously limit food choices for the rest of your life and to potentially limit social opportunities built around meals. For many patients, life after WLS means treating food as fuel, not as a source of drama, excitement, comfort, or a central life focus, that is, eating to live rather than living to eat. While some procedures may be reversible, for most patients WLS is a lifetime commitment, requiring a lifetime of major lifestyle changes.

4. Weight loss surgery can be dangerous. As many as 0.5% of surgery patients can die from the procedure, and up to 5% can experience debilitating medical complications.

3. It takes great bravery and strength to deflect other people's judgments and society's myths about obesity. Fat people are often blamed and shamed by family and friends with simplistic advice, unrealistic solutions, and uninformed prejudices. Whether it's for genetic or metabolic reasons or for diet and exercise reasons, willpower and discipline have never, by themselves, been enough. Our appetite regulators simply don't work. Without WLS, we don't know when we're full!

2. What gives anyone the right to judge which path is right for another? Is a person who runs a 10K taking a better or tougher route to wellness than the person who walks vigorously every day? Is working with weights better than water aerobics? Different strokes for different folks. Each of us finds our own way, and how dare others judge our path to health and longevity!

1. For many morbidly obese people, WLS may be the *only* realistic alternative for achieving a long, healthy life. The newest research provides irrefutable evidence that body weight is largely a function of genes—just like height or a family propensity for cancer. These genes help regulate appetite and metabolism. People prone to obesity seem to gain excessive weight easily, while finding it difficult or impossible to lose it.

Through Thick and Thin #18
(After the Surgery—6.5 Months)

Head Hunger and Emotional Eating

For the first time in my life, I know that I can trust the information transmitted by my stomach to prompt, stop, or otherwise regulate my consumption of food and calories. And yet…

Sometimes, even knowing that my body has all the nourishment it needs, I feel hungry. Or, more precisely, I experience what seem to be real hunger pangs, even when I know they're artificial. I call this "head hunger." My belief is that unless emotional eating is recognized, acknowledged, and dealt with, it can and will sabotage the extreme measures I have taken to live a longer, healthier life.

I thought about this recently when I spent a long night alone in a motel room during a business trip. When I travel, I prepare conscientiously to ensure that no matter the situations or unanticipated circumstances that may present themselves, I will have what I need to take good care of my body. In my former life (before WLS), when I found myself alone in a motel room, on the road, I used to stock the shelves with lots of sugar and other crap as comfort food to help me make it through the night. (After all, calories don't count when you're alone in a motel room, right?) Today, six months post-op and down 110 pounds, I've stopped buying those treats that used to assault my health and sabotage my eating plan.

But this night, I found myself preparing to repeat the pattern. I knew, with certainty, that I had consumed enough to meet my body's needs. And yet I felt an unmistakable hunger that sure felt authentic and demanding and deserving of a response. So I reverted and took two crackers out of a baggie.

In less time than it took to take that first bite, I realized what I was doing and *put both pieces back into the bag.* I became very clear, in that defining moment, that any apparent hunger messages I get when I know that I'm full are instead fraudulent, destructive, self-sabotaging *head hunger* messages. They are my habits, my patterns, my childhood, my unconsciousness about my body, and my past irresponsibility and unaccountability about my health.

I can binge on anything—even two crackers—if I eat when I know I'm full!

Putting something back uneaten—amazing! My life is really changing; my awareness is deepening; and I'm living, moment by moment and day by day, my commitment to using WLS to live healthy and long.

Head hunger is a message telling me that either I haven't yet done my requisite personal growth work to deal with and resolve all the emotional reasons I used to compulsively overeat, or that I presently have some more work to do. I invested years of my pre-WLS life on a searching and fearless journey of self-examination, therapy, and other personal growth work to figure out why I ate like I did and what I needed to learn, understand, or apply in order to change. And still, at times when I get too angry, lonely, or tired, I know I have more work to do. I need to remember to take good care of myself.

Through Thick and Thin #19
(After the Surgery—7 Months)

"Off the Rack"
or
From 4X to XL

I'm finally ready for my first bona fide post-op clothes shopping trip. I had repeatedly postponed what has always been a traumatic exercise in frustration and public humiliation. But I just couldn't make do with my old clothes any longer.

What an amazing difference 115 lost pounds makes! Contrary to my fears, my shopping excursion proved to be fun, exciting, inspirational, and successful. At thrift shops and Old Navy alike, I was reintroduced to three of the sweetest words in the world: off the rack! My new pants size, reflecting seventeen inches off my waist and 14.5 inches off my hips, has shrunk from fifty-six to a relatively trim forty-two.

As we shopped, and right in front of Kari's eyes, I transformed from a hurt little boy ashamed of his body every time he shopped into a "normal-sized" man who enjoyed looking at himself in the mirror and admired the reflection back. I am becoming one of "them"—those normal-sized people who, on some level, I have always both envied and despised.

Today I weigh what I did when I was married, a quarter-century ago. What amazes me is the difference between how I felt about my body and appearance then and now. The weights are about the same, but my self-perception has changed dramatically. Then, at 240 pounds, I felt fat, gross, repulsive, sluggish, out of shape, and full of self-blame and self-shame. Today, at just a hair under 240 pounds, I feel trim; fit; attractive; athletic; energetic; and bursting with self-esteem, self-pride, and satisfaction. My weight is the same, but viva la différence in my attitude and perception!

So last weekend, at a wonderful local music festival, I donned my new wardrobe and walked with a light spirit and a prance in my step. I drank in all the compliments, flirtations, and even all the blank looks of nonrecognition on the faces of those who hadn't seen me since my WLS. It reminded me of that vision I had long ago, seeing another thin man and feeling as if that could someday be me. Now it is!

When I was still morbidly obese, I told myself the story that I didn't really care how I looked or what others thought. My shopping expedition, new wardrobe, and public display of my new body now convince me otherwise. *I like looking good!* And that redoubles my commitment and my resolve to reach my goal and become so normal and average in appearance that I will never again have to deal with those accusatory looks and cruel comments. I'll never forget what it felt like to be fat, and my heart and spirit will always reach out to others struggling with obesity—but I'll never go back there. I enjoy being thin.

Through Thick and Thin #20
(After the Surgery—7.5 Months)

Exercise Is Not an Option; It's Now My Default

I reached a milestone—125 pounds off. I've now become one of "those people": I love to walk and move my body so much that I park at the far end of the parking lot and power walk to the entrance. I seek out opportunities to walk. Exercise has changed dramatically for me with my weight loss. Now that I can move without pain or fatigue, I love it for its own sake. And, of course, I love it for the way that it drives my continuing weight loss.

Exercise is no longer an option; it is my default. What I mean is that I am comfortably and naturally incorporating exercise into every day and into everything I do. I walk for fun and for weight loss and because it's become a joyful way to center myself and recharge my emotional, professional, and spiritual batteries.

My post-op blessings and joy continue to multiply exponentially. I still have some serious concerns and problems, but my *gratitude attitude* helps me reframe and cope with them. I see my doctor soon for a second endoscopy to check the healing of the ulcers. Until then, I'll appreciate and celebrate the boost to my accelerated weight loss that has resulted from my present inability to handle so many "normal" foods. I welcome the tradeoff: exchanging health for gluttony is serving me well. And I'm doing fine with an extremely boring and limited menu.

Through Thick and Thin #21
(After the Surgery—8.75 Months)

Getting Real About My WLS Problems

I've been doing some self-examination as I begin my ninth month post-op and add to my loss of 135+ pounds. I've renewed my commitment to being real about my problems with weight loss surgery. Getting real means acknowledging my gnawing frustration and irritation at the severe limitations upon *what* I can eat—not about the quantity of food I can consume, but the variety (or lack thereof).

The good news is my ulcers have healed. The other thing the doctor found was that my stoma appears to be the optimal size and didn't need any stretching. Some scarring and inflammation remain.

I was disappointed. I wanted a quick solution or magic bullet. I wanted the stretching of my stoma to suddenly make it possible for me to eat more than my bland, boring standard selection of foods. I hoped that henceforth I would be able to eat just about anything, only in small amounts and with a lot of chewing. It appears that's not to be the case.

Basically, my liquid/semisolid eating program doesn't change. I drink only water, with some occasional nonfat milk. I believe I'm averaging 500–800 calories per day. What I've *not* been able to eat includes: bread, anything with yeast/ flour/egg, salads, pasta, or most other things. When I eat anything not on my "OK list," I experience extreme digestive discomfort and then usually end up inducing vomiting to eventually end the discomfort. When I experience only mild discomfort, I go for a long and vigorous walk and that usually improves things.

I know that removal of my gallbladder imposes some digestive limitations. I understand (and am pleased) that my pouch hasn't stretched much, if at all, and that my internal staples are holding tight. Finally, I know that everyone reacts differently to WLS. But I very much want to know whether or not my present eating limitations are likely to persist, or whether they are likely to improve as my post-op time extends.

It certainly does seem that most of my post-op WLS colleagues have a much easier time of it. Most claim to be able to eat more things, in small amounts. And

I understand that those experiencing problems like mine are the least likely to talk about them.

I no longer have any doubts that I will reach my goal weight. I occasionally have concerns about continuing to lose weight after reaching my goal, but I figure that is a natural bit of distorted thinking and is mainly my fear and anxiety squawking.

I also have to admit that there's a big part of the smaller and leaner me that welcomes, even enjoys, the freedom and ease that I find in being confined to limited choices. I'm spared the necessity (and danger) of choice, even as I bemoan my loss of the dignity of it. For me, boring and bland can be wonderful and even liberating. While I insist on choices in every other area of my life, when it comes to food and eating, I really do like it easy and simple. Even during those terrible and counterproductive years of incessant dieting, my favorite was Stillman's, where if it was protein, I ate it, and if it wasn't, I didn't. Also, I recognize that for me, this tendency toward bland repetition is part of my transformation into a person who eats to fuel my body, not for comfort, joy, sensation, or fun.

Honestly, I treasure the tool of negative conditioning and reinforcement that has blessed me in my post-op period. I feel so terrible and awful when I eat things I can't that even starvation—and certainly monotonous blandness—is immeasurably preferable to feeling sick. And that, together with my restored appetite regulator from the surgery, makes it so much easier for me to ignore the emotional hunger and temptations that used to push me over the edge into compulsive overeating.

One of the best tools I've found and have used to neutralize my tendency to make myself the victim and the martyr is "reframing"—looking at a problem or situation from a different perspective, through new eyes—searching for the gifts contained within the difficulty. For example, if I couldn't join my family for restaurant meals because they served nothing I could handle, I could reframe the situation and turn that negative into a positive by walking around during their mealtime and seeing things and having adventures I would otherwise not have had.

And yet, I'm tired of social meals where I can't fully participate. I'm tired of needing to go for a walk every time a restaurant doesn't have anything I can eat. I'm tired of needing to bring my collection of safe foods with me when I travel. I'm tired of the constant stress and strain of keeping my body healthful with minimal resources. I'm tired of being so limited by circumstance, not choice.

And still, it is undeniably clear to me that all these frustrations and irritations are *nothing* compared with the health and fitness; the comfort; the freedom of movement; my improving appearance; and all the other joys, gifts, and blessings that my WLS has brought to me. But it is important to me—as a matter of principle, ethics, and integrity—that I be real about them, and share them.

Getting real about WLS doesn't mean trashing it or living like a victim or sitting on a pity pot. It simply means sharing the whole story—the positive and the negative—and never losing sight of the bottom line. A happy and healthy life will be the penultimate testimony to my WLS reality.

Through Thick and Thin #22
(After the Surgery—9.5 Months)

Shame, Blame, and WLS

Since my surgery I've been devoting ten or more hours a week as a volunteer e-mail coach to people who are considering weight loss surgery. One theme that continues to emerge is the shame and self-blame that WLS candidates almost invariably feel about their historic inability to lose weight "the normal way"—through diets, exercise, and sheer willpower. "Why can't I lose weight the way others seem to be able to do it?"

While I'm certainly no medical expert, I have become convinced through my process of WLS and recovery that confronting and disposing of this shame is one of the most vital pieces of emotional work that must be done before this tool can be used with optimal effectiveness.

I'm not sure if it's because I was simply carrying too much weight to deal with it incrementally; or if my metabolism slowed down and got stuck and nothing I could do would speed it up; or if my appetite regulator simply didn't work and never had; or if it's just the accumulated burden of a lifetime of blame, shame, hopelessness, and despair. But my experience is that for me, WLS was the *only* realistic alternative for achieving a long, healthy life.

To transform from a morbidly obese candidate for premature death into a healthy, active, fit man with a normal life expectancy, I needed a tool—weight loss surgery. And there's no shame in that. With a functioning appetite regulator—my still unstretched stomach pouch and my testy digestive system severely limiting my food and caloric intake—I've been able to do what had previously been both unthinkable and impossible. And once it didn't hurt to move, I've embraced a love affair with exercise. This has been my final proof that *it wasn't my fault all this time*! This has been the ultimate documentation that it hasn't been a matter of my deficient willpower, insufficient commitment, sinfully gluttonous appetites, or laziness. I had a medical condition that required a medical intervention and tool. I can now put my motivation and strength to good use. Now I'm almost at my goal, and, on top of the restored agility of my body, I feel so much lighter without the burden of the shame I had carried with me for so many lost decades.

Today, about nine and a half months after my WLS, I have lost 145 pounds. Yesterday was my annual physical exam, and my doctor confirmed that I no longer function as a diabetic, that I no longer suffer sleep apnea, and that I'm a very healthy and vigorous man, close to and rapidly approaching my goal weight. My blood pressure was a sublime 104/64, and all my tests confirmed my excellent state of health. In gratitude, today I began what will be a three-times-a-week program of weight training to further strengthen and firm up my body.

Through Thick and Thin #23
(After the Surgery—9.75 Months)

Dealing With Questions About WLS

I recently returned from my thirty-fifth reunion of my junior year abroad class in England. It was a wonderful opportunity to catch up with my dearest college friends and community. Most of the group had seen me at or close to my most obese (or had seen pictures of my former huge self on my Web sites) and they were stunned and congratulatory and asked an endless stream of questions about this strange and wondrous thing called WLS and how it had changed my life.

I had, of course, anticipated *the questions*. Living in a small rural town in the Pacific Northwest, sooner or later nearly everyone in town has witnessed my relatively rapid and amazing transformation from a morbidly obese man ("You'd be so handsome if only…, etc.) to an *invisible man*, approaching normal weight, average appearance, and blending in. Until my trip to England, I had been cautiously selective in what to share with whom. While I graciously accepted the congratulations and compliments, I choose to share my WLS surgery, experience, triumphs and struggles only with those relatively few dear friends and colleagues whom I trusted and loved.

I rethought this approach on the long, seemingly interminable flight from Seattle to London. So I was prepared for the onslaught of questions and fielded them with a distinctly different attitude and manner.

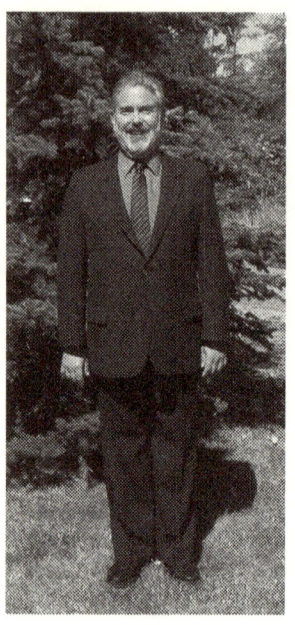

What ultimately changed my attitude and response to questions about my dramatic weight loss and transformed appearance was remembering when I suffered from obstructive sleep apnea. I had to sleep with a mask and a CPAP apparatus to force ambient air down my throat passage to keep it open and keep me breathing. For whatever reason—probably because I had already pretty much cast off my sense of shame about this particular medical condition—I decided, from the outset, to speak openly about my sleep apnea. I even initiated the discussion whenever people mentioned snoring, restless sleep, waking up fatigued, or any of the other indicators of sleep apnea. The result was incredible, and deeply gratifying: my sharing about my sleep apnea directly led several others to be tested in a sleep lab, where they were diagnosed with sleep apnea and got the medical device that had saved my life and may have saved theirs.

As I thought about the lives that were eased or saved by my openness about my sleep apnea, I quickly decided that it was important—my ethical imperative—to be just as freely open about my morbid obesity and subsequent weight loss surgery. For me, it was the right choice. Although none of my classmates were morbidly obese, virtually *everyone* had a friend or family member who was, and who had given up on ever restoring their health, comfort, and vitality. My hope is that every time I share openly and candidly, the upsides and downsides, about obesity and WLS with others who are respectful about these topics, I just may be setting into motion a chain of events that may help those who are still suffering find help and hope. Seeds are planted.

So, at my reunion, I made the time to answer fully and honestly questions about every aspect of my WLS and post-op recovery. Why did I choose such a drastic intervention? What were the risks? How painful was the surgery? How long and difficult was the recovery? How expensive was it? Why can't I eat normally now? Why am I always drinking water? Why do I walk instead of taking a taxi in London? How has it affected my energy levels and my work life? How has it affected my sex drive and sex life? How has it affected my relationships with my wife, family, and friends? How do I socialize without centering the interaction around food? What about diarrhea and constipation? Will I waste away to skin and bones after I've reached my goal weight? What does it feel like to wear clothes off the rack again? Knowing what I know now, would I do it all over again? Is it appropriate for morbidly obese children and teens?

I returned home with a new attitude and behavior pattern when it comes to answering questions about my weight, surgery, and body. I still don't spill my story with everyone who compliments me on my appearance. But when I sense that people are genuinely curious and will be respectful in hearing my story, I share it. I'm always sure to give a balanced presentation of the pluses and minuses. And I feel so good knowing that my openness may prove to be the key that opens the lock that has been shackling a brother or sister of the scale.

Through Thick and Thin #24
(After the Surgery—10.75 Months)

Vows Kept and Challenges Met

I made myself a solemn promise one year ago when I decided to have my weight loss surgery. It was a vow that, at that time, I couldn't imagine being able to keep. I promised myself that by the end of my first summer after WLS, I would complete a legendary and demanding ten-mile hike through old growth forests to the Pacific Ocean and back. I intentionally set this very ambitious goal, because I had a great deal to prove. I wanted a challenge so unthinkable and impossible in my pre-operative state that its eventual achievement would really mean something. It would mean that I had used the tool of WLS to totally change my lifestyle, dramatically improve my health, and attain an unprecedented level of physical fitness and mobility.

I just returned from my hike, joyful and triumphant! Besides being beautiful, invigorating, and fun, it proved to be a powerful metaphor for my recovery from weight loss surgery and the miraculous transformation I have experienced through this process.

The walk was difficult and, at times, scary. It was also exhilarating and empowering. The first 3.5 miles was on a beautiful trail through the giant trees in the temperate rain forest. I was grateful for a warm, sunny day. The path was a boardwalk, raised above the sometimes wet and muddy land, and the steps moved up and down to match the contours of the ground below. The length and the elevations were comparable to my daily walk, so I walked briskly and finished the first phase in less than an hour. At the very end of this link, when the path moved sharply downhill to the beach and surf below, I encountered my first moments of doubt and panic.

I should explain that I departed on my hike with two internal voices battling for predominance within my head:

- *Maxi-G (maximum weight Glenn):* the "I can't do it" voice of my old, morbidly obese and mobility-impaired self—was resigned to failing again.

- *Mini-G (goal weight Glenn):* the "I can do *anything*" voice of my new, healthy, and fit self—was ready, hopeful, even confident.

The steep descent to the shoreline plunged Maxi-G into the familiar trap of fear. If the drop to the beach is so steep, he worried, how will I ever be able to handle the ascent back up? Mini-G reminded me that this fear was a phony issue, a distraction, and that after months of climbing hills I was more than ready to deal with the challenge. I heeded his advice and carefully climbed down to the beach, savoring the moment.

Actually there wasn't much of a beach. That presented the second opportunity for Maxi-G to stir the pot. I had planned the hike to arrive at the shore at low tide, because the park service had cautioned that at high tide this three-mile second leg of the journey could be impassable and dangerous. I had expected to trek along a flat beach. It soon became clear that I would need to walk offshore on the now exposed rocks and tidelands until I picked up the return trail three miles south of my arrival point. The rocks were slippery, and I have balance/vertigo problems anyway, so this was another unanticipated challenge. Because I had to constantly walk away from the shoreline to round the next in an endless series of points of land, the supposedly three-mile jaunt morphed into a four- or five-mile ordeal. But the vista was magnificent, and the isolation splendid, and once I was able to stifle Maxi-G's complaints and whining, I had the time of my life. It took three hours to negotiate the tidelands and find the return trail.

By that time, I was finally and fully ready to leave Maxi-G behind. I'm pleased to tell you that I abandoned Maxi-G—and his negative sabotaging voice of pessimism, despair, and limitation—in that pristine spot, and there he will remain forever. Mini-G lives on, peacefully and alone, within me.

I walked the three-mile final leg back on the boardwalk and through the woods at an accelerated and ener-gized pace, feeling lighter without the burden of Maxi-G's voice. I was now certain that I would complete my challenge in grand style.

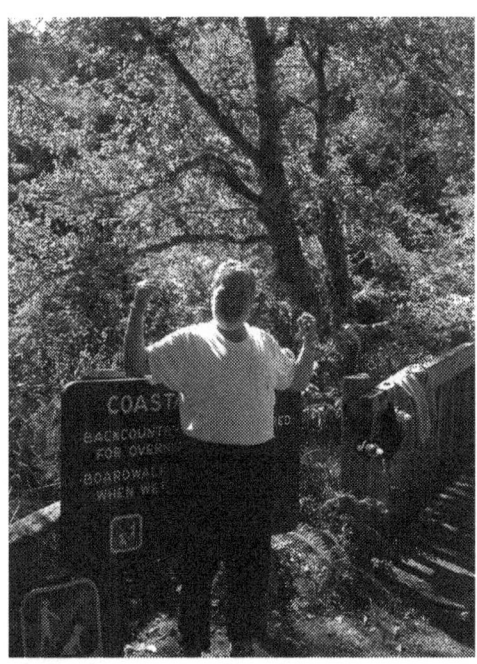

It was wonderful and somehow fitting, that about a mile before the end of the trail, I encountered a group of hikers. One of them was a friend I hadn't seen since before my surgery. She didn't recognize me after my 150+ pound weight loss, and certainly didn't expect to see the sedentary, lethargic Glenn she remembered hiking so vigorously on the wilderness trail. It was a timely reminder that I'm no longer the man that I once was, neither physically nor spiritually.

At trail's end I celebrated, yelling and pumping my fists in the air, and I noted, with great pleasure, that I felt like I could walk another mile or two or five.

As I drove home from my adventure and the hike that was metaphorical for my liberation from the oppression of morbid obesity, I felt a deep inner serenity. I kept my vow; I met my challenge. In the process, I proved to myself—on a deep emotional, gut-feeling level that is totally distinct from my head knowl-edge—that my pre-WLS inability to lose weight and gain mobility was not a product of some internal character defect, or insufficient commitment or will-power. I proved that I am whole, and I am powerful, and my commitment and will can change my world and create the life that I want.

4

The Man I've Become

Through Thick and Thin #25
(After the Surgery—11.5 Months)

Distorted Body Image, Distorted Thinking

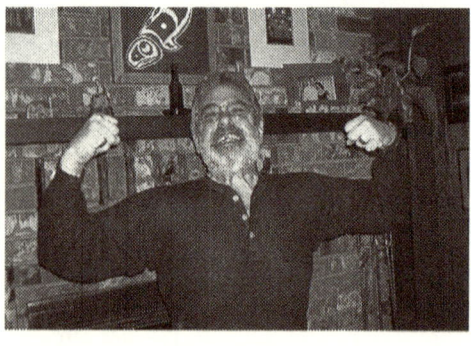 My mind can be such a strange and puzzling realm! Sometimes my perceptions are as sharp, focused, and precise as a laser beam, cutting to the essence of a situation or finding the solution to a problem. Other times, especially when it concerns my body image and issues, I'm surprised at how grossly distorted my perceptions can be.

These days, eleven months after my surgery, I'm experiencing problems getting a realistic and accurate sense of the dimensions and boundaries of my new, post-WLS body. I've lost 160 pounds (the equivalent of a "normally sized" person that I've been hauling around for most of my life), and I'm sometimes very confused and just plain wrong about my size and shape.

The distortion seems to work two ways. First, I'm continually surprised by how fat I still appear when I examine recent photographs. The scale and clothes labels reassure me that I have never weighed less, at least since my adolescence. But, to myself, I still look fat and swollen. It's not my vision growing dim; it's a legacy from almost a lifetime of conditioning that I was a fat and disgusting pig, skin stretched tight over several hundred pounds of ugly fat.

It's almost as if, when I look at a current picture of myself, my glasses automatically shift to a distorting prescription that displays a body mass that's no longer there. Exercising every day, and subsisting on very little food, I *feel* so thin and light and trim. That's why I am so surprised, and disappointed, when my image on film still looks so outsized to me.

Actually, it's not so surprising after all. This is the kind of toll that years of listening to and believing negative self-talk can take on a sensitive and vulnerable spirit that has internalized the *shame*.

At the same time and alternatively, I find it quite ironic that I can't quite seem to get a handle on how relatively small and lean my body has become. I'm amazed every time I feel the emergence of another rib or muscle in a place that had been a fleshy, gushy soft spot for so long. Although I know in my mind that I now wear size large in men's clothing, I continue to be incredulous every time pants or a shirt in that size actually fit me. My mind is screaming "Don't even try; it will never fit; you're wrong again about your size; you're still too fat" every second that I'm trying on the clothes. It's not until I zip and button the pants that I realize that this is what it must feel like when clothes are tailored just for me. Doing the laundry, I dangle my 36–38 underwear and can't quite get it that this tiny garment is large enough to contain my girth.

When we're doing home repairs or rearranging furniture, I still find myself waiting for Kari to squeeze into the thin corridor or constricted space because my inflated self-image won't fit, although my body is now actually smaller than hers. Last weekend while visiting dear friends, I spent five minutes trying to figure out how to best climb into the bed that was wedged into a corner, before I realized that I was now slim enough to walk around the bed. I just can't get used to being the flexible, mobile person *who can*, after so many decades of being the stuffed, immobile person *who cannot*.

I'm hoping that, with more time in my new body, I'll become better adjusted and find the self image that is just right for the man I've become. I also hope that I'll never stop savoring the glorious anonymity of being an *invisible man* in public: no one gawking at me because of my girth; no more pity or harsh snap judgments in the eyes of the people that I pass on my walks. Sometimes, it feels so good just to melt into the crowd.

Through Thick and Thin #26
(After the Surgery—12 Months)

Out of the Closet

On this anniversary, I've been remembering how my life was before surgery, comparing my life today, and marveling at the transformations. One of the most surprising changes is that today, at my goal weight, I'm boldly striding "out of the closet" with the astounding revelation that I'm a *clothes hound*! This is about the last thing I would ever have predicted for my life after WLS.

It turns out that I've been telling myself a fictional story all those *fat years*: that I just didn't care much about either my appearance or my wardrobe. The plainer, more shapeless, the blacker the better: baggy sweats whenever I could; ties and jackets only when there was no other option, and even then ties were loosened at the first opportunity and jackets came off soon thereafter. "I just don't care about vanity, appearances and such trifling contrivances as clothes," I convinced myself. All these years and it now turns out that I was telling myself a whopper of a lie.

Now that I *can* and *do* look good in nice clothes, I find that I actually love dressing up. I love the feeling of wearing clothing that is colorful, fashionable, form-fitting, and elegant. I love making an entrance into a room. I savor the feelings of confidence, power, and attention that accompany my choice of attractive clothes. I like wearing suits, jackets, ties, turtlenecks, tight jeans, horizontal stripes, outrageous colors, and everything else that painful experience (and my mother) taught me to avoid. Today, I take great pride in my appearance, knowing how hard I've worked for it, and just how much I've sacrificed to create this new body and look.

I chose to have my weight loss surgery because I wanted to live a long and healthy life. Everything else was just an added benefit and afterthought, the "gravy" in my old food-centered way of thinking. I never would have guessed that it was only the intense power of my denial that had convinced me that clothes and appearance and pride and confidence—or even my comfort and self-esteem—weren't, in and of themselves, important enough to justify my weight loss surgery. Today, I know different and I know better.

Through Thick and Thin #27
(After the Surgery—13 Months)

Falling Off the Wagon and Getting Right Back On
or
Beware of that Slippery Slope!

The other shoe finally dropped. It wasn't until the last two weeks of my first year that I slipped and "fell off the wagon." It's not like I started eating like a madman, like my former self. It was more a matter of getting sloppy, taking things for granted, and relaxing what had been, until then, my 24/7 vigilance. By the time that I was restored to a state of full consciousness, I had gained back five of my 160 pounds so painstakingly shed during my first year post-op.

In the clarity of hindsight, I can see clearly how I stepped off my path. First, I must admit that I sometimes indulge in a bit of self-pity, albeit as briefly as I can manage it. While 100% of WLS patients experience some kind of limitation on the foods they can eat and tolerate, I'm one of what seems to be a fairly small minority of WLS-ers who are *severely* limited in their food choices. Most days I do pretty well with accepting what I can't eat, and enjoying what I can. In many ways, I find the limitations on my choices to be a comfort and relief, and I do well with boring and routine. It helps me focus on the *fuel*, and disengage from the *food*.

Unfortunately, over the course of the year, I've discovered a few naughty treats that even my testy tummy will tolerate. And so, from time to time, I've indulged in my own customized version of the dreaded soft calorie syndrome. In the weeks leading up to my long-anticipated first WLS anniversary, I reverted to the kind of celebration that led me to my health crisis, morbid obesity and weight loss surgery, granting myself one of these treats most nights.

Second, around the same time, the weather in the Pacific Northwest turned cold, wet, and uncomfortable. Again, I cut myself some slack, and shortened my daily outdoor mega-walks.

That's all it took: a few hundred extra calories a day consumed; a few hundred fewer calories a day burned. Simple math—and the difference between continuing my weight loss and pursuit of my ideal weight (so close now!) and starting to put it back on.

The good news is how I responded when I figured out what had been going on. I wasn't even tempted to blame and shame myself, or to extend my vacation from vigilance. I immediately stepped back, observed myself, and shifted into action. I logged and limited my caloric intake, going back to the eating plan that had worked so well for me and brought me to this point. I lengthened and ratcheted up my daily workouts. I cleansed my house of the treats. And voilà! As if my magic, the extra pounds hurried off, and I've resumed my losing ways.

The episode scared me, but it also offered me some precious gifts, starting with humility and the slap-in-the-face reminder to stay awake, stay aware, and stay off of the pity pot. I also reaped the thrill of successfully using my new tools and strategies to first stop, and then remedy, my setback. And I feel so strong, proud, and assured because I turned it around and now know that I *can*, whenever I must.

This was a very cheap lesson, and I'm grateful for it. I gained confidence for my future by climbing right back onto that proverbial wagon and driving on full-speed ahead. *I know now, in a way that I never did before, that I will never again slide back into obesity.*

Through Thick and Thin #28
(After the Surgery—13.25 Months)

From Lowered to Great Expectations

Now that I'm close to my ideal weight, I'm really enjoying shopping in thrift stores. Recently, as my pile of clothing possibilities grew, Kari and I suspended the process long enough to explore my obvious exhilaration and the reasons for it. What emerged surprised and sobered me.

My words cascaded out. I shared how incredible it felt to absolutely *love* every piece of clothing I selected. How much fun it was to be able to wear stripes, spots, bright colors, and everything else that I had been taught to shun, on penalty of embarrassment and humiliation at looking even more fat than I was. I reminisced yet again about the ordeal it had always been for me to go shopping for any piece of clothing. I gushed on and on about how different and thrilling it was now to expect clothes to fit and to look terrific on me.

Kari reminded me, with the understanding and wisdom she always manifests, that the clothes shopping experience should be entirely about picking only apparel that I really treasure. I say remind, but actually I never knew this.

Talking it out, I realized that I've spent my entire life as a clothes consumer carrying around awfully low expectations with respect to what I had the right to have. I was so focused on bravely and cheerfully accepting bland, styleless, shapeless, ugly clothes just because they fit (more or less), that I never even considered the concept of being entitled to choose clothes that I loved. So it was a revelation for me to realize that I had definite tastes and preferences (like horizontally striped shirts and tight, form-fitting jeans, instead of those baggy, boxy monstrosities I wore all those years.)

My explosion of insight didn't stop there. I started taking stock of all the other areas of my life where, as a fat man, I expected and accepted, with appreciation, so much less than I was entitled to enjoy. I was flooded with memories, most bittersweet, about all the times, in all the domains of my life, where the story I told myself was that it was OK with me to be left out or get second-best once again. It was a painfully disturbing story of sadly and terribly *lowered expectations*.

So many times and occasions—growing up, in my relationships, at work, and at play—I felt that second-class status was the best that someone like me could expect. Like the time I couldn't join my daughter on a horseback ride because the stables had weight limits—or all those amusement park rides or exciting physical adventures I couldn't join—or the jobs or relationships that could never be. I put myself "one down" and everyone else "one up" because I was fat and they weren't. How much have I held myself back in my life because my expectations were so low, because my self-worth was so impaired?

The good news is that today, I love, accept, and value *all* aspects of my self—mental, emotional, spiritual, and physical—and I have such *great expectations* about what I deserve! It's not just clothes that I treasure, but also a relationship that thrills me, a right livelihood that fulfills me, and a life that I love. And I finally know that's not asking too much.

Through Thick and Thin #29
(After the Surgery—15.25 Months)

Obsessing on My Oral Compulsions

My mouth craves constant action, stimulation, and movement. I derive great joy and satisfaction from the kinetic energy inherent in chewing, sucking, or otherwise mouthing things and substances. My oral fixation began before the reach of my memory, and has continued, unabated, in the fifteen months since my weight loss surgery. I haven't let my oral compulsions interfere with my post-op eating plan. However, I still find myself struggling to understand the origins of my oral cravings, and to find healthy alternatives and replacement behaviors—or at least minimally harmful things and substances to keep my mouth satiated and out of trouble.

It's amazing to picture myself at work a decade ago. In those ancient days I'd be displaying a stunning sampler of compulsive behaviors and implements at my desk. I'd have a cigarette in one hand, a caffeinated Diet Coke in the other, and an array of thoroughly chewed pens, pencils, straws, toothpicks, and other useful oral tools scattered across my desk, alongside snacks, rolls of mints, and packs of gum. I worked and lived compulsively, I ate obsessively, and my mouth was always full of something.

Over the years, as I did my emotional work, I began to understand bits and pieces of the origins of my oral obsessions. I came to see that the circumstances of my childhood and my shame about my obesity (and my inability to change it) had dug a huge hole in my soul, and that I was desperately trying to fill that spiritual void with food, soda, smoke, and chewable goodies. Later, I learned that *nothing* could ever be enough to fill that hole unless and until I forgave myself, reached a state of peace with my parents, and really and truly started believing that I was a good human being and "enough." I was able to quit smoking, wean myself off soda and carbonation, and greatly improve my eating program. But my oral fixations persisted.

My parents are both deceased, so it's impossible for me to deconstruct my childhood. However, it seems likely that I was never breast-fed, and I know for sure that my mom was uncomfortable with cuddling and displays of affection. Maybe that's where this all started. I'll never know. And I guess, in the final analysis, I really don't need to know. I've come to believe that, at some point, it's less important for me to understand the origins of my oral compulsion than to find ways to live with it, without hurting myself or threatening my new fit and thin state of lightness of being.

Harm reduction has been my primary strategy to prevent my oral cravings from sabotaging my WLS and post-op recovery. I have continued my constant mouth kinetics, but now I'm sucking, chewing, and/or swallowing less harmful substances than junk food, soda, smoke, and pens. My water bottle has become a part of my anatomy, and I drink that life-sustaining blessing constantly throughout my waking hours. Once I was far enough out from surgery, I began sucking on mints (always paranoid enough about swallowing one to make sure it fully melted in my mouth). They worked well to satisfy my cravings and to impart a pleasant taste in my mouth, but before long a handful of mints a day turned into too many. They were practically becoming one of my food groups, and I was terrified to find myself declining opportunities to eat protein to offset the extra calories consumed when I devoured a full container each day. So I switched to another brand of mints, which, for some reason, melted slower, lasted longer, and never tempted me to binge.

The good news is that, for today, I can live a healthy life and maintain my weight loss even with my obsessive, compulsive consumption of water and sugar-free mints. But I would love to find a way to live in peace and serenity without needing my mouth to be chomping every waking moment. These behaviors aren't threatening my health, but I still find the twin demons of shame and blame bedeviling me every time I notice how hard, and sometimes impossible, it is for me to "just be."

Through Thick and Thin #30
(After the Surgery—16 Months)

Fixing My Fixations II

I really want to understand the roots of this particular compulsion because both me and my mouth are getting tired of this nonsense and wasted energy, and I resent the loss of control and power over my own body parts and functions. I don't want to continue engaging in old behaviors that no longer serve me or promote my health and inner peace. So I asked a special friend who is also a very gifted and spiritual psychoanalyst for his off-the-cuff insights into my oral imperatives.

Apparently, Sigmund Freud had a lot to say about these compulsive behaviors. He observed that in response to anxiety or stress, some individuals regress to the earlier oral stage of their life when they gained such pleasure and security from nursing at their mothers' breasts. Freud believed that an individual acting out their oral fixations is feeling needy and dependent on others to meet those needs. Freud also identified a second related oral phase, the oral biting stage. As I understand it, he believed that the individual who reenacts their biting preoccupations from infancy is making the statement: "I'm in need *and* I'm angry. My needs are not being met. I want what I want, and I want it *now*!" One of his successors, Erik Erickson, slightly reframed oral fixations as being about people expressing their anxiety and issues around trust and dependency.

Hmmm…feeling needy. Feeling dependent on others to meet my needs. Feeling angry because they're falling down on the job, and thus my needs aren't being met. Impatience. Trust issues. Is it a coincidence that so many of my personal life issues and challenges seem to center around issues of trust and issues of frustration and impatience when others disappoint me or don't follow through, and thus I'm not getting my needs met? I think not. As one of my teachers and mentors, Elizabeth Kubler-Ross, used to say, "If you believe in coincidence, you're just not paying attention!" Well, I *am* paying attention, and I do want to figure this one out.

I have so many questions, and so few answers, that I've decided to try something rather dramatic to first understand, and then to free myself from my elusive and potentially self-destructive oral obsession. Here's what I've decided to do. Starting now, I am going to refuse to chew, lick, suck, bite, or otherwise use mints or any other substances or implements—other than bona fide food, beverages, and medications that are a regular part of my daily consumption. I'll do this for one week, two weeks, a month, or however long it takes to get to the bottom of this mystery.

Since I clearly use my mouth in this fashion as some kind of deep-rooted response to feelings of anxiety, stress, distrust, and abandonment, I figure that whatever demon or genie or other surprises that are usually kept distracted by my oral activities will find some way out. They will reveal themselves to me in some form—and I'll be keeping a hypervigilant watch to see what feelings or responses arise when I refuse to sacrifice my self-will and power.

I've successfully used a similar approach to deal with *head hunger*—that phantom appetite coming from unresolved feelings that makes me feel hungry when I know that my stomach is full. Instead of eating, I'll go for a walk, explore what I'm feeling, and then usually find or deconstruct the feeling that is disguising itself as hunger. Once I can name it, I can claim it, and that fear, anxiety, or feeling loses its power over me. I'm hoping that this similar strategy will help me understand—and finally resolve—the unseen, unknown forces that drive me to keep my mouth in perpetual motion.

Through Thick and Thin #31
(After the Surgery—17.5 Months)

Making Peace with My Mouth
While Bringing My Heart up to Speed

Within a few days of beginning my oral abstinence experiment, I found the answer I had been seeking all these years. Why do I obsessively and relentlessly pop things into my mouth?—*Because it's a learned behavior that became a habit.*

Although I was expecting feelings and emotional storms to erupt once I stopped my nonsubsistence chew-a-thon, the main things I experienced, and only then for the first few days, were feelings of boredom, emptiness, and a lack of taste, excitement, and stimulation. Nothing more. I didn't experience any suffering or deprivation or withdrawals. I wasn't tempted to eat or drink more. There was no deep secret, only long-ago learned behaviors that I had never tested. Once challenged, they melted away.

Here's what I've concluded about *my* oral fixations as a result of the experiment.

- My oral fixation is a learned behavior. Sometime long ago, for reasons that have long since disappeared, I learned that mouthing and consumption behaviors provided me with comfort, excitement, and stimulation—the illusion of filling up that bottomless unworthiness pit within me (my "I'm not enough hole"). It felt good, or postponed my feeling bad, so this learned behavior worked for me, and I continued to work it. It became a habit that persisted long after both my need for self-comfort and its initial apparent effectiveness receded.

- My learned behaviors can be unlearned. All I had to do was try. When I suspended the habit, there was no deep, ultimate truth that emerged, or any replaced behavior that demanded reinstatement. Another one of the stories I'd been telling myself all my life—that chewing on things helped me feel better—proved to be an empty lie and illusion. I was amazed, and delighted, that I didn't have to pay any dues or penalty for stopping the habit that virtually took me over, but delivered no real payoff. In the future, my first step to challenge any other self-sabotaging or nonproductive learned behavior or habit will be to just stop it—and then to notice the results.

- I have a compulsive, addictive personality, and consequently I will compulsively devour anything that stimulates or occupies my mouth *and* that I make readily available to myself. If I don't have these temptations around, I don't miss them, crave them, or seek them out. If I have them close at hand, I do, and I will consume them. Just as I don't keep unhealthy foods in my home, I will no longer keep gum, mints, and their ilk in my home. Maybe I'll splurge on mints on a business trip, or a long drive. But my home is my temple, and I only want to keep healthy things in my temple.

- If I've been held hostage to a learned behavior/habit relating to mouth candy, what other learned behaviors or habits in other domains of my life are unnecessarily holding me back or hurting me? I plan to munch on that question for a long time.

Still abstinent and continuing the experiment, I felt light-headed while taking my morning walk. I ended up in the emergency room, diagnosed with bradycardia (slow heartbeat). Although my heart was strong and undamaged, something was wrong with the electrical timing mechanism, and so my heart was pumping too slowly. As a result, my brain and organs weren't getting the oxygen and nutrients they needed. A pacemaker was installed two weeks ago, and now I'm feeling healthy and energized again.

I realize that if I hadn't had weight loss surgery and lost my excess weight, this heart episode could have been dangerous and even lethal. There was no connection between my slow heart rate and my WLS (more likely it's a genetic endowment from my maternal side of the family). But because I am now thin and fit, I was spared what could have been a very serious and debilitating health crisis. You can imagine how thrilled and proud I was, even in the midst of my hospitalization, when after the dreaded treadmill test of my heart's capacity, the doctor told me I had the healthy and strong heart of an athlete. How sweet is the aftermath of WLS.

Through Thick and Thin #32
(After the Surgery—18 Months)

I'm Still the Same Man

My wife and I don't do a lot of group socializing. Kari has struggled to deal with the ravages of chronic fatigue syndrome for more than fifteen years now, and even when she has the energy to socialize, the cacophony of voices, fragrances, and sheer kinetic energy at a party can devastate her stamina. Also, I've learned to savor my own, and our own, quality alone time, and to prefer small, intimate settings and conversations over large parties. The food and eating limitations imposed on me by my testy tummy also discourage us from participating in social situations planned around food.

So I was a bit anxious, on several counts, last Friday evening when we attended our first real dinner party since my WLS. As we drove to the affair, I noted in passing that I had never met any of these folks before, which meant that they had no idea of my former state of morbid obesity. I wondered, with a mix of curiosity and mild concern, how they would see me and how I would feel under their gaze.

It was so strange—and also exciting and powerful—when I walked into the host's home, was introduced to the very charming couples assembled, sat down to chat, and realized that I *was the thinnest person in the room*! I don't know why this should have been so surprising to me, but it was. And I felt this unusual and pleasurable satisfaction in knowing that, unless I brought up the matter (or unless we played strip poker and I lost badly), none of them would ever know, or even suspect, that for the first fifty-four years of my life I was usually the *fattest* person in any gathering.

The next morning—exactly eighteen months after my weight loss surgery—I participated as a delegate in the U.S. Presidential Caucus. I'm not going to get into politics here, but suffice it to say that I lined up for a chance to address the 500 folks in attendance to share my personal perspective on several issues.

I wasn't nervous at all about what I wanted to say, but I *was* a bit anxious about my presentation. I've been an outspoken advocate for various causes my whole life, and have done so many press interviews, presentations of testimony at legislative hearings, and conference presentations that I have no fear about what I say. But I had always assumed that the source of my power as an advocate or speaker was directly tied to my (former) sheer physical bulk. I wondered, as I waited to speak, if my words would be received differently, or have less impact, coming from a man of more normal size. Surely there was a significant risk that my transformed size and shape would reduce the "weight" of my arguments.

I need not have worried. It was gratifying to see and really understand that my physical bulk had *never* been the true source of my personal power. My remarks were well-received, and I thanked my Higher Power again for this validation that *who I am is not defined—or even affected—by my bulk.*

If I had been paying closer attention, I would have already internalized this understanding. Several months ago, when I co-facilitated my first seminar since my surgery and weight loss, my co-facilitator expressed surprise that nothing about me had changed, except my weight and appearance. She had expected, on some level, that the transformation of my body would correspondingly change my feelings, my actions, my self-presentation to the world, and my spirit (i.e., who I really was). I wasn't ready to hear and accept her feedback then, but now I know it to be true.

Eighteen months post-op, I now know the following three things are true.

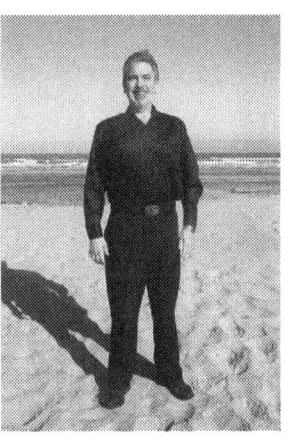

- I'm the same person now that I was before.

- I struggle with the same problems and issues now that I struggled with before my surgery, with the notable exception that weight loss is no longer a concern.

- My weight loss surgery was one of the most powerful acts of self-love I have ever experienced.

Contrary to my life-long paradigm and misunderstanding, weight doesn't make the man (or woman). I didn't decide to have the surgery because I didn't like who I was; I had the surgery because I *did* like myself, and wanted more life to live. Today, my reflection in the mirror truly matches who and what's always been there. The critical difference is that now everyone else can see that too.

Through Thick and Thin #33
(After the Surgery—19.75 Months)

Stretching Comfort Zones
or
As I Shrink, I Redouble My Efforts to Grow

As I continue to reduce my weight, and solidify and redefine my lean muscle mass, I'm discovering more and more opportunities to stretch my comfort zones with respect to the physical activities and adventures that my normal weight now permits. I've lost 100% of my excess weight (180 pounds), so physical challenges that were inconceivable to my former fat self now beckon me to partake.

In recent months I have experienced the joys of trying formerly impossible pursuits. I've learned that it's just as important for my personal growth to keep testing and stretching my comfort zones (i.e., the things I feel comfortable, excited, and reasonably confident about) as it was for me to tackle the difficult task of losing my excess weight.

I've always operated on another core belief and personal rule—that whenever an opportunity presents itself to me that makes me feel anxious or resistant, I *must* try it. I've found that what I resist persists. I choose to take the risk and, hopefully, reap the rewards and push a bit farther the boundaries or limits I place around my own life. Thus, in recent months, I have either sought out or accepted the challenges to:

• Sea-kayak for the first time in my life for 20+ miles through the pristine islands and icy waters of northern British Columbia

• Spend a day socializing (at a safe distance) with grizzly bears and their young

• Participate in an Elderhostel Big Band Camp that helped me grow musically and improve my jazz improvisation and sectional Big Band playing, on both my clarinet and alto sax

Each activity was—in its own way—both an intimidating and ultimately joyful challenge. I'm already adding to my list of other challenges I want and intend to try in order to continue my personal stretching in coming months and years.

• White-water river rafting

• Salmon fishing

- Sailing

- Parachuting and paragliding

- Water skiing

- Horseback riding

- Walking in a marathon or half-marathon

- Going back to school and relearning the musical scales and chords after a 40+ year break, which will help me elevate my jazz improvisation

- Jamming at several improv nights at local music clubs

The truth, which I sometimes resist and sometimes accept, is that in my new and improved body and shape, I can do just about *anything* I choose to try. It's taking me lots of time—and unlearning and relearning—to see that I need not use my obesity as an excuse for opting out of life's abundant challenges and opportunities. The story I told myself for most of my life—*that I can't*—has been exposed as a lie. I'm working hard to take responsibility and accountability for extending my comfort zones as wide as they can reach.

I'm convinced that using the WLS toolkit to lose my excess weight is only the first of an endless array of second chances I'll get to re-create my life and redefine my limitations. There's nothing more satisfying to me than checking off another "stretch goal" and thereby expanding my Universe, experience, skills and capacities, and dreams of what could yet be.

Through Thick and Thin #34
(After the Surgery—21 Months)

The Gift of WLS Support Groups

Last night was the first time in a while that I've been able to attend the local weight loss surgery support group. I'm so glad that I went. It was gratifying to see how the group had grown, diversified, and matured during my absence. It was thrilling to witness the transformation of all these big-time losers who had been pre-op or early post-op the last time I saw them. One after another, they shared their stories, challenges, experience, strength, and hope, and that is, of course, what support groups are all about.

My reconnection with my WLS support group reminded me what a precious gift these gatherings can be. Cofounding the group was initially a self-serving act; that is, I craved and needed face-to-face access to the pioneers who had walked the path, and blazed the trail, for the rest of us to follow. I must have brought twenty-five questions to the first meeting—and I left with most of them answered. More importantly, I left with the validation and confidence that I too could and would use the WLS toolkit to get healthy, live long, and prosper.

I attended the support group faithfully for my first year post-op, and then, having reached my weight loss goals and harvesting the energy burst I experienced in my slimmed down body, I stopped going. Life just got busy, and since weight was not the central issue anymore, other things took center stage.

At the meeting, however, I was powerfully reminded of all the *other* reasons to attend, besides meeting my own needs.

- being there for others, just as so many veterans were there for me in my time of need

- sharing proven, practical tips and strategies for dealing with the various problems that test and frustrate newcomers

- remembering where I used to be, how far I've come, and how important it is to keep working my food and exercise programs so that I never take a step back toward the morbid obesity that tortured my body and soul

- feeling again the very special and unique bonds that WLS-ers feel and enjoy with each other

Our discussions were easy and comfortable, and our laughter flowed like the fast-moving stream near my home. We laughed uproariously about things that only a group of fat people or formerly fat people would "get"—like the challenges we experience(d) with various bodily functions. When some of the women in the group started complaining (and laughing) about how tough it can be for fat women at intimate times, we men regaled the group with our own counterpoint stories. Everyone was encouraged, acknowledged, applauded, and heard. No one was put down, excluded, disrespected, ignored, or abandoned. It was clear that everyone was there to help and to support. That's why WLS support groups are such a blessing and gift for so many of us.

Through Thick & Thin #35
(After the Surgery—23 Months)

My Weight Stays Stable, but My Shame Keeps Resurfacing

Today, as I write, I'm at my ideal weight, and I continue to be able to make sufficient minor adjustments in my caloric intake and caloric burn to maintain my weight stability. I just wish that I could find some magical way to exorcise the sense of shame that continues to resurface every time I experience any kind of health-related problem or crisis.

Seven months ago I became faint while walking and soon was informed that I needed a pacemaker. It was clear that this medical condition was genetic in origin and had absolutely nothing to do with either my previous morbid obesity or my weight loss surgery.

Then three months ago, again while walking, I started feeling dizzy and light-headed. I almost fainted, as the world whirled around me in a maddening state of vertigo. I was tested for inner ear and hearing problems, but the tests revealed no problems. A brain CAT scan was done and revealed some calcification in my carotid arteries. Again, this condition is common in people my age, regardless of their weight or weight loss, and hopefully soon will be treated and resolved so that I can resume the vigorous daily exercise that has become a treasured and very special aspect of my inner and outer life. Since my surgery, my cholesterol has been at levels I used to dream of, and my heart remains strong and undamaged.

What was so interesting—and disturbing—about both incidents was that the very first place my mind and emotions went was to my shame. It's the same shame that burdened my spirit every day I walked this earth as a fat man. I did a great deal of therapeutic work about my feelings of unworthiness before my surgery, and I continued this healing work post-op.

In my naiveté, however, I made the dangerous assumption that now that I was a man of "normal" size and weight, I had finally and successfully completed my lifelong struggles with both obesity and the accompanying feelings of shame, humiliation, disgrace, and personal dishonor.

I was mistaken. It appears that I have internalized my sense of shame so deeply and profoundly that whenever *anything* goes wrong with my body, I immediately accept that the cause is my years of gluttony and obesity. I take total responsibility and feel completely accountable for causing my corporal calamity. I don't question; I blame myself. I don't seek other explanations; I punish myself harshly. These feelings have nothing to do with physical reality, but they have unfortunately become an ingrained part of my interior emotional landscape. This is a pattern I want to break, but I now suspect it will take much longer to lose the shame than it did to lose the excess weight!

I do reasonably well in both my professional and social domains when my words or actions are questioned, challenged, or attacked. I take a quick, searching, and fearless moral inventory of my attitudes, actions, choices, and behaviors. If I did something wrong or unkind, I take responsibility for my misconduct, make amends, and do my best to clean up my mess—and to learn from it. At the same time, if I become clear that the conflict is all about the other person (or the situation) and not at all about me, then I let go of anxiety, guilt, and bad feelings and move on, clean and confident.

It doesn't work as simply or as well with respect to my own physical problems. I continue to drag around the terrible weight of unjustified personal dishonor until my wife talks me through my delusions. I want to underscore my new understanding and belief that *fat shame* can be a self-sabotaging adversary that may relentlessly try to undermine your confidence and successes long after weight issues have been managed.

This is one vicious circle I am aching to break. Apparently some of my psychic wounds—originally, but no longer linked to my weight—lie so deep and hidden that they still defy detection and remedy. I've admitted to myself, reluctantly, that I have more interior work still to do.

Through Thick and Thin #36
(After the Surgery—24 Months)

My Bottom Line

It was two years ago today that I had my vertical banded gastroplasty.

According to my medical team, I would probably have been dead by now without my *weight loss surgery*—and its matching gifts of my 180-pound weight loss, and my transformed body and lifestyle. That's my personal bottom line as I look back upon the path that led me to this day and milestone.

The promise of my bariatric surgeon, Dr. James Weber of Seattle, has been kept. I've reaped the *precious prize* he promised me if I scrupulously followed his instructions, kept moving my body, and totally changed my relationship with food.

On this day, I've been reliving and remembering every step and setback along the way. I've been reminded of my pre-op fears and anxieties (Was I making a fatally wrong choice? Would I fail yet again?); the challenges of the surgery itself and the agony and suffering of those difficult first weeks and months of post-op recovery; and the severe continuing limitations on my food choices.

My outcomes—being more fully alive than ever before, living once again in my body, the extraordinarily improving my mobility and energy, and looking and feeling great—confirm that I made the right decision for me. They also underscore my personal bottom line on weight loss surgery: it saved and extended my life. I feel blessed, grateful, and so joyful!

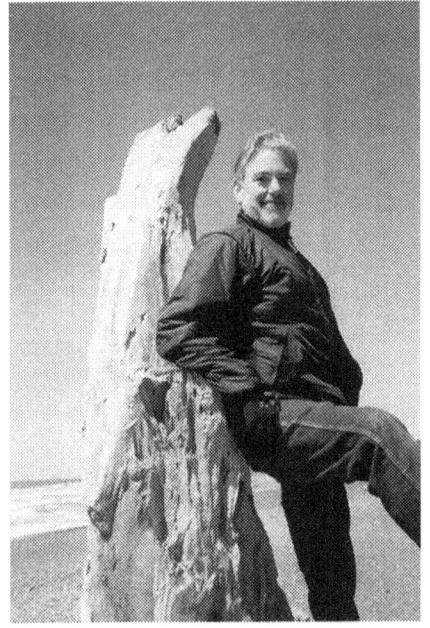

In the distant past I would have celebrated this special occasion by treating myself to a fabulous feast of food. Today, I choose to celebrate my achievement by taking one of my long and favorite hikes through the old-growth temperate rain forest near my home. Afterward, Kari and I will enjoy a hot tub together, build a roaring blaze in the fireplace, and review the photographs that chart my path from desperation to exhilaration, from sickness to health, from fat to thin.

Weight loss surgery is a difficult choice to make, and it's not for everyone. It requires an extraordinary depth and consistency of commitment, strength, courage, and perseverance. It often requires a network of supportive partners, family, and/or friends. It requires deep emotional work and a lifestyle transformation. It is most assuredly *not* a quick fix or an easy way out of the horrors of morbid obesity. But for me it's been a true blessing.

PART II
Every Body Is Different

Seven Other People Share
Their WLS Stories

5

Chub-Chub

by
Pam Davis, RN, CCM

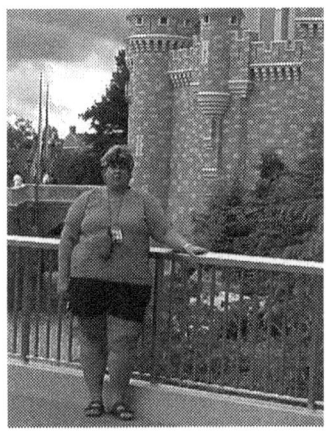

"Good morning, Chub-Chub." And so it began. Thirty-three years ago at my first day of school, that is how I was greeted (by the cutest blonde-haired, blue-eyed boy I'd ever seen). My initial response was, "Hi." I was so happy he had spoken to me. Then it sank in...that phrase at the end...what he called me. *"Chub-chub." I had never really considered myself fat until that point.*

I was greeted the same way, every day for the next twelve years. As he grew taller and cuter, I grew taller and fatter. Now don't get the wrong idea. I was not morbidly obese in high school. Not even close. I was 5'8" and 170–180 pounds in high school (oddly enough, only a few pounds more than my current weight, which I am so proud of—the weight at which a few angels even refer to me as thin). But as a teenage girl growing up in the "Marsha, Marsha, Marsha" 70s and the "Material Girl" 80s, I was always one of the fattest girls in my class, and that hurt.

Everyone else was wearing the Levi's with the little tag on the back that showed your size 3, 5, 7, and there I was, stuffed so tightly into a pair of 13s that I literally could not sit down. I pulled my shirt down to hide that shameful double-digit number. At this point, back-to-school shopping consisted of a 1 1/2-hour drive to the nearest Lane Bryant (and in those days, their clothes were not the beautiful hip styles they have today).

I'm not one of those people to blame all my problems, including my weight, on my parents. *But* it didn't help that the moment school was out for the summer my mother would put me on a diet, stating, "You'll lose all that weight over the summer and then when school starts back, you'll be a whole new person."

I always wondered what (besides a few extra pounds) was wrong with the person I was.

To this day, if I think too long about grapefruit juice I will start gagging. That was a recurring diet theme at our house. I can remember one summer being on a diet and feeling like I was starving to death, so when we went to the grocery store I hid in one of the aisles with a jar of Jif peanut butter. I took the lid off and scooped it into my mouth with my fingers as fast as I could. (I may be the reason those foil seals now cover the jars! My apologies to the grocery store in Horse Cave, Kentucky, and to any unsuspecting customer who got home with "my" jar of peanut butter).

Thinking about it now, I truly don't know how I got so big and my parents did not. My mother is only 5'2" and has always been about twenty pounds overweight. Daddy was one of "those people"—the ones with the metabolism such that at church homecomings or family reunions he would eat three full plates of food and one full plate of dessert. We lived on a farm for several years, and going out to eat once or twice a week was a treat, not the daily occurrence it is for many people now.

I can count on one hand the times I ate cereal as a child. Breakfast was typically cinnamon rolls or biscuits and sausage. My favorite days were after we had killed hogs, and Momma would fix sausage all day, as we had to taste test until it was seasoned just right. Even toast was a bad thing—each slice of bread had four pats of butter and then was sprinkled with cinnamon and broiled. The rest of our meals were normal farm-type food: meat loaf, fried chicken, pork chops, vegetables cooked with fatback. Of course, they were still vegetables so I did not eat them. We made homemade ice cream once a week during the summer. We lived so far out of town that fast food was not the culprit. I played on the tennis team for two years in high school, rode my bike at home, and I was not a couch potato because we didn't have cable, and video games were not around. So *what* was my problem?

There was one fabulous summer when I was fifteen. I had lost some weight and was feeling pretty good about myself. I had on the cutest little pink shorts outfit, and we were all hanging out in the Pizza Hut parking lot. A guy a year or two older was there. He had had a few, and he made the mistake of calling me a fat bitch. Before I knew it, I had slugged him. I learned then that if I reacted when people called me names, I just drew more attention to myself, and I never changed their opinions or biases anyway.

During my junior and senior years of high school, my daddy became very sick with leukemia and lung cancer. My mother was gone ninety miles away to be with him at the hospital, and I was burning up the road. By then we had moved to town, and I was working full time (3–11 PM) at the local Jerry's Restaurant, featuring free meals when you worked. There was Wendy's, Pizza Hut, and Long John Silver's all in a row! Now with my own car, money to buy food, and very little supervision, I became a *wild child*! At the ripe old age of sixteen, I could drink most of the guys in my class under the table.

I was the one the guys wanted to hang out with, but not go out with. (I should add that in our senior year of high school I invited five different guys to the prom and, of course, was turned down by all of them. Self-esteem? "I don't need no stinkin' self-esteem," I told myself.) During my senior year, my daddy died. By summer, I had moved into my own little apartment, where I had free reign on eating. My weight started its upward climb, although at the time, I was still hovering around 180–190 pounds.

I met my future husband at a keg party in a milk barn. (Give me a break. It was rural Kentucky in the winter. What else did I do?) We got married in May 1985. At that point I was about 190 pounds, wearing sizes 14–16 and sometimes 18. We lived on a farm, and he worked hard all day. I wanted to prove I could be a good wife, so I cooked every recipe I had learned in four years of home economics: homemade yeast rolls, chocolate pie, fried chicken, fried pork chops. His job relocated us to Massachusetts in 1987.

After three months, I learned I was pregnant. I had free reign to eat again, but this time for two! I didn't know anyone. I worked days, and my husband worked nights. It became my habit on my way home to stop at one of the marvelous Greek delicatessens and get a foot-long grinder, onion rings, and, of course, the baklava. I also kept chocolate doughnuts in the house at all times. I would sit at one meal and think about what I wanted for the next. I gained seventy-five pounds; my son weighed 9 pounds, 8 ounces. The day of delivery I weighed 272. My weight went down to 230 before I became pregnant again. This time I had morning sickness and only gained thirty-five pounds; my son weighed 10 pounds, 9 ounces.

Stuck in what seemed like a foreign country—alone with two small children while my husband worked all day—I ate. I am embarrassed to say how many times I would bake an entire cake from scratch, eat about half to two-thirds of it, and then throw the rest away because I didn't want my husband to know I had eaten that much of it.

He was (and is) so supportive. My husband has never said anything to me about my weight. The bigger I got, the more supportive he was. He has always said, "I don't care what size you are, I married *you*, not a size." Honestly, while part of my brain thought, "Cool, I can keep on eating!" the other part thought, "What's wrong with you? Why don't you care? Don't you see how gross I look?" Because I wasn't working and didn't really know anyone, I didn't feel any pressure to lose weight. I kept thinking, "I'm not going to worry about my weight until it affects my health." At this point, I was twenty-five years old with no health problems yet and weighed around 250 pounds. (Hello, size twenty-four!)

Finally, in 1990, we were able to transfer closer to home. We have now called Tennessee home for fourteen years. We have raised our children here; I've gone to nursing school here; we have friends here; *and I got my life back here.*

In 1991, I started nursing school. I came home the first day excited to tell my husband I was neither the oldest nor the fattest person in the class. (I had been seriously worried about being both.) After the first year, I decided to try Opti-fast. (Oprah, you little ol' inspiration, you!) Actually, it wasn't just Oprah who inspired me. As a nursing student, I had to educate my patients. I felt like the world's biggest hypocrite every time I had to haul my big ol' butt into a room to teach someone about a diet (kind of like the Marlboro man showing you how to apply a nicotine patch).

Let me just say this: the combination of consuming only five ninety-calorie shakes a day, raising two toddlers, and going to school full-time resulted in more than a little bit of stress. Honestly, I do not know how my husband put up with me! Talk about being in a terminally foul mood. Ask any nursing student and they will tell you: school is stressful. Combine that with no food, and it's a wonder I didn't knock over a McDonald's and bury my face in the French fries.

I had been drinking Opti-fast shakes every day for three months when I reached my breaking point. A group of us had been studying for exams. They had ordered pizza and I just snapped as I was mixing my orange shake. No more shakes! I started eating that pizza and, I swear to God, all sixty pounds I had lost came back the next morning. But, that little bit of weight loss gave me a taste of something I yearned for—cute clothes! I was down to a size eighteen before going off the Opti-fast plan.

After graduating from nursing school in 1993 and starting work, my weight was around 250 again. The parking lot at work was right beside the university's athletic track. At least two or three times a month I would get to work early and walk around the track, thinking, "This is it!" This is the time I'm going to stick with an exercise program. Then, every time, reality crashed my party, and I disappointed myself again.

I was working at my first real job ever, and a lot of overtime was available, so there was no time for exercise. We ordered out lunch nearly every day. ("Steak-out, anyone?" "Sure, and don't forget the large sweet tea and chocolate cake!"). Then on my way home I passed nearly every fast-food restaurant known to humankind.

I didn't want anyone to know the sheer volume of food I could consume, so I started a few new tricky little habits. On my way to work each morning I stopped at the doughnut shop and got two doughnuts and two pigs-in-a-blanket ($5), which I ate on my way to work. We ordered out nearly every day for lunch ($8). Then, on the way home from work, I'd stop at Krystal, Taco Bell, or Wendy's ($5) and eat my *first* supper. Then when I got home I'd eat my *real* supper with my family. It hit me one day that I was spending about $20 a day on food!

I decided it was time to spend that money on getting rid of my excess weight. Fen-phen (fenfluramine plus phentermine) was not dispensed in Tennessee. I had to drive to Kentucky. Three different times I went on fen-phen. I lost weight every time. (As I recall, I lost fifty pounds and put about sixty back on; then lost the sixty pounds and put about seventy back on; and the last time I lost seventy-five pounds and put it all back on.) Fen-phen worked, but only while I was on it. On that now-known-to-be dangerous drug combination, I really wasn't hungry (such a foreign concept). Since I wasn't hungry and didn't have cravings, it was easy to eat healthier. It made sense to me—at least it did at that time.

Being a nurse, I monitored my blood pressure every week while I was on the drug, and, to my knowledge, my heart valves survived intact. I should also mention that I worked in a surgical intensive care unit and had taken care of several open gastric bypass patients. At the time, I thought that surgery was only for really old, really sick, really fat, fixing-to-die people. Many of the nurses I worked with were overweight. (None of us considered ourselves *obese*—what a horrible-sounding word.) We went back and forth, we'd all diet, and then we'd all give in and order out. There still wasn't any peer pressure to lose weight, and my husband remained supportive. We were both working so much overtime and were so tired, it was just easier to go out to eat.

By 1999 my weight was at 300 pounds. I had continued my mantra of "I'm not going to worry about my weight until it affects my health", and I continued to wonder who on earth had to buy those size 28s at Lane Bryant? Well, by the year 2000, I had my answer on both counts.

First, I went to Lane Bryant to buy a pair of jeans to wear on casual day. The size 28s didn't fit; they wouldn't even fasten. I had to buy a pair of size 30 jeans. I was in a state of meltdown! In addition, I was now on two medications for my blood pressure, which still ran in the 160s over the high 90s to low 100s, I was on Vioxx for pain in my heels, and I was on medication for gastroesophageal reflux disease (GERD). Thank God, it was only GERD; I originally thought I was having heart palpitations.

I was then at a job where by 9 AM we had our lunch order ready to go! I started to notice that about an hour after eating my shoulder hurt. That suggested I had gallstones. When I saw my doctor, and she confirmed I had gallstones, I read my growing list of physical ailments on the paperwork I carried to the front desk: gallstones, hypertension, GERD, morbid obesity. What an awful sounding disease!

The day I was sitting at my desk (after eating a Captain D's lunch) and I could hear my pulse pounding in my head, it finally hit home. If I don't do something, and soon, I'm not going to live to see my kids graduate high school, much less college. Without question, my weight was now adversely affecting my health. The question then became, what am I going to do about it?

I was in the car on my way to see the surgeon about my gallbladder when I heard an ad on the radio for laparoscopic gastric bypass surgery. When I arrived at the surgeon's office, I asked him about it. He said that, while he didn't do the surgery, he thought I was an excellent candidate for it, and that my gallbladder problems could wait until I could check into weight loss surgery. I made an appointment to attend the next WLS seminar.

My husband and I attended the seminar late in January 2001. I was very impressed by the program coordinator—she had had open gastric bypass surgery several years before and lost more than 100 pounds. She looked great. We met the surgeons that night. I took my paperwork home, filled it out, and faxed it back the next day.

My husband was not sure at first. He was at work, discussing the seminar and expressing his doubts, when a co-worker told him that she had lost her excess weight after gastric bypass surgery. She answered his questions and alleviated his concerns. After that, he was convinced.

It took me a few days to gather the information they needed from my doctor and to get it to the bariatric clinic. My insurance company, United HealthCare, received the request on Tuesday morning. On Thursday morning, the case manager called me and asked for my date of surgery—my request had been approved!

We scheduled my surgery for March 2, 2001. My husband went with me to see the surgeon. I was very impressed. He was direct, straightforward, and very nice (not a quality that every surgeon possesses). I had already talked with another surgeon I knew who performed gastric bypass surgery and asked about his doing my case laparoscopically (with a minimal incision and intrusion). He told me he wouldn't even consider it because of my size. I asked this second surgeon if he thought he could do me "lap." He explained that what limited him was the length of the instruments, and that with my body mass index (BMI) of 53, I was at a higher risk for needing an open procedure.

Then he said what every woman yearns to hear (especially in front of her husband), "Stand up, and let me see how your fat drapes." Now I knew he was seeing if I was an apple (harder to do "lap") or a pear (easier to do "lap" because there is less fat high on your abdomen). I knew all this, but it still didn't make it any easier to hear.

He said he thought I could be a candidate for a laparoscopic gastric bypass. I told him all I wanted was for him to try; if I had to be converted to an open procedure, that would be fine, but I wanted to give it a try. He explained that I would be only his second laparoscopic gastric bypass patient and asked if that concerned me. Being an intensive care nurse, I explained that typically I was not worried about the surgeon nearly as much as I was worried about the anesthesia. We confirmed the date for March 2, 2001. I was told several times, "It's just like getting your gallbladder out." I now had *two weeks* to get ready for surgery!

I should add that I'm a huge Tennessee Titans fan, and, while watching the Titans vs. the Ravens, I saw them introduce Tony Siragusa for the Ravens (one of those players that Titans fans loved to hate). His weight was 330 pounds, the same as mine. That really hit home and helped me decide I was doing the right thing. I had to get rid of that weight. I was the size of a professional football player!

During those days leading up to surgery, I didn't have a lot of "last meals," as some people feel compelled to do. We did go to Macaroni Grill the Sunday before surgery. I ate so much of the bread, Italian nachos, and pasta that I barely had room for a bite of dessert.

It's true that sometimes we nurses think we're pretty smart. We know how things work (or at least we think we do) and sometimes we decide we can improve them. I knew I was *supposed* to be on clear liquids on Thursday and drink my magnesium citrate that afternoon. Well, my rationale was that if I went on full liquids, such as tomato soup, Monday, and then did clear liquids Tuesday, Wednesday, and Thursday, there wouldn't be that much food in my system for the magnesium citrate to work on. I wouldn't be up all night in the bathroom. *Wrong!* Not only was I still up in the bathroom all night, by the time I got to the hospital I had lost seventeen pounds! (At first I thought that was a plus, *but* the rest of the story is that I was so dehydrated that they had to give me a ton of fluids in surgery, and I wound up having to have my wedding ring cut off because of the swelling.)

In between bathroom runs that evening, I was sitting on the couch with my husband, and it hit me, looking at him and the boys, that this could be the last night I would ever spend with them. I started thinking, "You are making a conscious decision to be put to sleep and have an elective surgery that is not an emergency. Anything could happen." My mini panic attack hit—swift and hard—but blissfully, it passed quickly.

I thought back to that day when I was sitting at my desk and thought about not living to see my kids graduate. I confirmed my choice. I admitted to myself that without surgery, I was going to die young, and that this surgery was the only possibility I had of losing enough weight to have a healthier and hopefully longer life. I hugged and kissed my boys that night, told them that I loved them, and prayed that I would come home to them. I did.

Now, before I go into some of the details of my hospital stay, please realize that I love my surgeon and I love the hospital where I had surgery. I'm sure that the minor problems I experienced happened because it was a new program, and I was one of the first to go through it. I only mention them here because I used those incidents to make sure those issues wouldn't happen at *my* bariatric clinic—and so that other clinics developing WLS programs would carefully consider and address these concerns from a patient's perspective.

I arrived at the hospital and was placed in the videoscopic surgery area. The nurse came in to take my vital signs with a regular blood pressure cuff. *Honey, I weigh 330 pounds: don't you think you might just need the large cuff?* Unfortunately, no large cuff was available, so my pre-op blood pressure couldn't be recorded. We tried a thigh cuff (it looked like it was made for Moby Dick), without any better results. Since I *had* (notice the past tense) hypertension, they decided I needed to go back to the holding room and get an arterial line so we would know my blood pressure.

Six attempts later, I didn't really care if I even had a blood pressure, much less what it was! Although they kept giving me drugs, I was still very much aware of all six sticks and how each one hurt like blue blazes. Once in the operating room,

I will never, ever forget that the program coordinator was standing there at my side, holding my hand when they put me under. No one will ever know how much that very simple act of kindness meant to me.

Several hours later, I remember being in the recovery room and seeing the surgeon. I managed to croak out, "Did you do it lap?" He said that he did, and that he now knew he could actually have done someone quite a bit larger laparoscopically. That pleased me greatly.

I made it to my hospital room around 8:00 PM. After all that "it's just like having your gall bladder out" business, I had told my husband that he could just go on home after I got in my room, that the kids (eleven and thirteen) would be alright at home until he got there, and that they could just come see me the next day. Let me just say that after many rounds of nausea in recovery and finally arriving in my room, I let him know very quickly that he wasn't going *anywhere*! Of course, bless his heart, he had figured this out hours before I did and had already made arrangements for the kids to go to a friend's house for the evening.

The next morning, the surgeon came in and asked me how I felt. Well, I couldn't point to a single spot and say, "This hurts." Instead, I felt intense soreness all across my abdomen. I felt as if I'd done about 800 sit-ups. He told me I would be going down for a "swallow" to make sure I didn't have any leaks. This guy who looked like he was all of twelve years old picked me up in a bariatric wheelchair. (I freaked out: that wheelchair was huge; I felt like I was sitting on a deacon's bench.) He took me to radiology, handed me a huge (8–12 ounce) cup of contrast medium (after tasting it, I have always referred to it as *liquid crap*), and told me to drink it.

Now, I'm not a rocket scientist and I was under the influence of Demerol, but if my stomach now only holds 1/2-ounce, exactly how am I supposed to drink eight ounces of crap? When I asked him that, his answer was "Just drink it." Okay, apparently I had to draw him a picture. I said, "I had gastric bypass surgery and my stomach now holds 1/2-ounce; you've given me at least eight ounces to drink. Now do you see the problem I'm having with this?" He responded, "Just drink what you can." After about four or five swallows, I thought I was going to barf, so I told him I couldn't drink any more. He said, "Fine, just hop up here on the table on your stomach." I looked at him as if to say, "Are you on drugs?" I wasn't hopping anywhere! I asked whether it was okay for me to lie on my stomach after having major abdominal surgery. His response was that it must be, because my doctor ordered it. Never one to be shy, I told him I wasn't moving anywhere until my surgeon told me I could.

Well, God love him, not two minutes later my surgeon came to see what the problem was. I explained that I had serious doubts about the age and mental capacity of the radiology tech, doubts about the amount I had to drink, and worries about lying on my belly after surgery. He told me it was okay to lie on my stomach; we had to do that to get the test completed. The test took about three hours "because I couldn't drink enough." *Uggghhh, if I ever meet that technician in a dark alley...!*

Anyway, I got back upstairs, and guess what. The test was negative! All right! I'm thinking water, Jell-O. Well, the water came, but it had methylene blue dye in it, another precaution to check that I didn't have a leak in my new pouch. That was another drink that tasted like crap. I sipped on one cup all night. The next morning they brought me two more because I hadn't been able to finish the initial cup of it—ughhh. I went to the bathroom and my pee was green (a sign that the dye had made it through my system). The nurse came in, and I announced that "My pee is green, my drain is red, and I'm not drinking anymore dye!" (Gee, who'd want to be my nurse?)

The surgeon said that was fine: it was obvious I had no leak. Yeah! It was time for the good stuff: blue Jell-O, regular water, and broth. By this time I was feeling better. I was getting out of bed and walking around the unit on my own. By the third day after surgery, we were all waiting for that life-altering event: the first post-op bowel movement, which is *the* sign that one is ready for discharge. My hubby had gone back to work; I was getting back and forth to the bathroom by myself. I went to the bathroom and ta-da: a bowel movement!

Then it's time to get up and wipe. Hmmm. Let's see, if I lean back and reach that way—nope, that didn't work. Let's try to lean over and reach under—nope. After about fifteen to twenty minutes of standing up and sitting back down, I decided there was no way to get there from where I was. I had to give in and pull the emergency cord in the bathroom. By the time my true angel of a nurse arrived, I was sobbing. She came in there and must have thought I'd fallen from the way I was acting. She said, "What's wrong? What's wrong?" I managed to sob out, "I can't wipe my butt." She gave me "the look" (the one reserved for teenagers when they say something totally out there) and said, "Is that all? I thought you were in here half-dead." I was still sobbing. "But I'm a nurse. I shouldn't need you to have to come wipe my butt." Again came that look and reassurance that it was truly no big deal. Then she clinched the deal, "Guess what? You get to go home now that you've had your bowel movement." I had totally forgotten about that part! The very *best* part!

I'm here to say that the first week home after surgery was *hard*. I had to remember that if this were easy, everyone would be doing it. The first day after I was home, I must have seen every fast food commercial known to man. I had my Jell-O and my broth. The next day, it seemed like every station on the TV was advertising the new Dairy Queen fried chicken salad (some silly Big Bird–looking thing). I had to go to the bathroom, took off running (not easy after surgery), and didn't make it in time. I was sitting on the commode, head in hands, crying. My husband came in there to see what was wrong.

"Why on earth did I have this surgery?" (Actually, knowing me, it probably came out as "Why did *you* let *me* have this surgery"?) "I can't eat right, I'm hungry, I can't even make it to the bathroom in time, and what have I done? Waaaaaahhhhh" (imagine a Lucy Ricardo type of whine about now).

God love him, my husband held my hand and asked if I remembered when they told me there would be days when I felt like this. No, I didn't. Well, okay, maybe I did. *Crap, I hate it when he's right.* A couple of days later (bathroom issues resolved), I was hungry. I called the program coordinator and explained that apparently the surgery didn't work on me. "I'm hungry. I thought the whole purpose for having this surgery was to not feel hungry, and I'm hungry. Do you hear me? I'm hungry!" She very patiently explained that water, broth, and Jell-O weren't going to fill up anyone no matter how small her stomach is. *She also explained that the surgery was on my stomach, not on my head.* It was going to take my head a few days to figure out that no, my throat hadn't been cut—I just wasn't taking in as much food. I think she also might have mentioned that I should get up off the couch and stop watching the TV with all those hateful commercials on it. Hmm….

I started a new job on March 19, 2001, a bit more than two weeks after my gastric bypass (bad timing, I know). It was hard. My brain felt like being back at work, but my body wasn't yet convinced. I was so tired. I can still remember taking a shower, and, by the time I was finished, I was too tired to dry off. I had to lie down wet on the bed and rest. That so-called sluggo effect lasted for a while. I like to blame it on the anesthesia. Truth is, it was many things: anesthesia, narcotics, but mostly the fact that my body went from consuming 3500+ calories a day to less than 400–500, and it was in hibernation mode. I knew it would pass, but in the meantime, I had to make myself get up and get moving.

The day of my surgery, I weighed 330 pounds. (They stopped one of my blood pressure medicines while I was in the hospital, and my GERD was gone with the act of the surgery.) I lost thirty pounds in the first month, seventy-five pounds in three months, and 100 pounds in my first six months post-op. There went the other blood pressure medicine! Then, over the next year, I lost my other sixty pounds and reached a low weight of 170 pounds. I then stabilized somewhere between 173–178 pounds.

It pleased me when people at work who I had never really met would ask me how I had lost my weight. I loved to explain to people about the surgery and how much better I felt. I kept a pile of my surgeon's cards at my desk, and distributed quite a few. It was so strange when some friends and co-workers didn't recognize me after my weight loss. I look at some of my "before" pictures, and, while obviously there is a difference, I still see "me." I must say that I have a lot more doors held open for me in my new body!

However, there was one disturbing aspect of achieving dramatic weight loss. Some of my friends were very supportive and constantly wanted to know how much I was losing until I became smaller than they were. Then, things magically changed, and they didn't want to hear about it anymore!

One of the truly great things about the hospital where I was working was that they had a wellness center on site. They oriented me to the equipment, set up a weight training program, and even monitored my pulse the first few times to make sure I wasn't overworking myself. I started going there regularly about a month after surgery. When I first got on the treadmill, it was at two mph. (I felt like someone's granny.) I would love to say that I went five days a week every week. The truth is I didn't. (To all patients reading this, do as I say, not as I did.)

The truth is that I always have, and likely always will, hate to exercise. I would go for four to six weeks, then slack off for a few weeks, then start back, and then slack off. Finally, I started thinking about having plastic surgery and wanted to make sure I was in good shape for that. That's what really motivated me to work out. I was really focusing on the weight training aspect and was developing great muscle tone. (Of course, one would have to dig through the excess skin to find the muscle, but it was and is still there.) For Mother's Day this year, I asked my husband and kids for tennis rackets to help me get back in the "exercise is fun" mode. It has helped some. I like to play tennis, but I suck at it! Oh well, chasing the balls is exercise too, isn't it?

I have found it is so important for me to be an active participant in a support group before and after surgery! Before surgery, the only concept I had of a support group was seeing AA meetings in the movies. As soon as I attended one, they became such an overwhelmingly positive thing—everyone sharing their successes, their setbacks, and their milestones. Aside from following the eating guidelines my program gave me after surgery, I have to say that my participation in a support group was the best thing I could do to help myself be successful after surgery. Actually, research has shown that patients who participate in support groups long-term have better outcomes than those who do not.

Notice that I said a support group, not a "bitch and moan" group. (Some are more of the latter than the former.) A support group will give help through the tough times. My husband and boys were supportive of me at home, and my co-workers were too. Friends and family have also been a valuable resource for me. This doesn't mean, however, that one shouldn't have surgery or can't be success-ful without a supportive family or circle of friends; it just means that some may have to find or create their own source of emotional and other support through groups or other vehicles (e.g., online).

I had maintained my weight at 173–178 pounds for the last two years, and then thanks to a kidney boulder (too big to be a mere stone) that kept me nause-ated and in pain for about a month this summer, I've lost another ten and I now hover at 165–168.

The only thing I take now (in addition to my vitamins) is Clarinex for aller-gies (required if you live in Tennessee) and Nexium for ulcer prevention. *I am happier, healthier, bolder, prouder, and louder than ever.* My only regret is that I didn't have surgery sooner.

Now that I am 3 1/2 years postsurgery, my eating is pretty normal. When I go out to dinner, the only difference between me and anyone else is that I don't drink while I eat. That is still the hardest part for me. I used to drink three to four glasses of tea or Diet Coke with every meal. They warned me after surgery to stop drinking 30–45 minutes before eating (so my pouch would be empty and could hold the food I would eat), and to wait at least an hour after eating to start drink-ing again (so I didn't empty out my pouch too soon, which can result in increased hunger and too little absorption of the nutrients in the food).

The other lingering effects from my surgery (besides weight loss and saying good riddance to my comorbidities) are a permanent lactose intolerance and a continuing experience of *dumping syndrome* (acute nausea, pain, and other symp-toms). Some patients never experience dumping syndrome; some only experience it for a period after surgery; and some, like me, have it long-term. Actually, I have grown to *appreciate* dumping syndrome. It provides me with negative reinforce-ment when I eat something I never should have eaten in the first place!

My dumping syndrome episodes appear to have no rhyme or reason. One time a couple of bites of sugary stuff goes down fine; the next time I'm assuming the fetal position on the couch with a cold rag on my head. Actually, I think it's that fear of the unknown that keeps me pretty straight. It only took one time driving down the road at 50 mph and experiencing dumping syndrome to make a believer out of me! My son had just gotten a chocolate chip cookie dough milk-shake from Jack in the Box. He was raving about how good it was. *"Come on, Mom, just take a sip."* I took two swallows. It wasn't even five minutes before I thought I was going to die right then and there in the van. We crept home and by the time I turned the van off, he had to help me in the house. Trust me, there is no ice cream anywhere on this planet that could ever be worth enduring that feeling again.

Head hunger is another of the legendary pitfalls of weight loss surgery. Early on in my recovery, there were times when I thought I was hungry even when I knew, with a certainty, that my pouch was still full. I knew this for sure because I had just eaten an hour ago and hadn't had anything to drink. I would physically look down at my stomach and say out loud to myself, "You *cannot* be hungry; you just ate an hour ago! Forget it; you're not getting any more food." It worked then. I need to use this routine less and less often as my recovery consolidates.

Weight loss surgery is a tool (just like a cordless screwdriver is a tool). If one doesn't read the owner's manual and follow the directions, one cannot expect an optimum outcome. Of course, the reduced pouch size will induce some weight loss, but not the maximum positive benefits.

I got my priceless tool for permanent weight loss on March 2, 2001, and since then I've created my own owner's manual. I have committed myself to following the *tool rules* forever:

- *Eat my protein first and half of every meal.* (Eat good, lean, high-quality, dense, nutrient-rich protein. Think chicken, fish, and beans, not sausage, bratwurst, or mini-corndogs!)

- *Drink a minimum of sixty-four ounces of water a day.* Recent research shows that for every twenty-five pounds you're overweight, you should add an additional eight-ounce glass of water to your total consumption.

- *No snacking or grazing.* Period, never, end of story. Once it's allowed the first time, those old habits start right back.

- *Exercise daily.* Move more today than you did yesterday, and tomorrow, move even more.

- The only truly *forbidden forever foods* are sodas or any carbonated beverage; and *avoid* (not eliminate, but avoid) pasta and rice, sugary foods (which lead to dumping syndrome), and high-fat foods.

I'm convinced that if I follow these rules forever, I will keep off my excess weight. I followed these rules scrupulously, and within eighteen months after surgery, I had lost 160 pounds. I went from 330 pounds, a BMI of 53, and a size 30–32 with hypertension, GERD, and pain in my heels and knees to 170 (now at 165 pounds) with a BMI of 25, wearing size 10–12, and no longer suffering from hypertension, GERD, or pain.

The best things about life after WLS are getting rid of all those medicines; being able to bend over and tie my shoes; shopping at the mall or wherever I want; being able to play basketball and tennis with my kids; and looking over my shoulder to see what is taking them so long!

Yoo-hoo, Oprah, Dr. Phil! Did I take the easy way out? What do you think?

I challenge anyone who thinks that *weight loss surgery* is the easy way out to follow me or any other WLS patient through the process. (I would also challenge the medical directors at the 1-800-Hell-No companies to do the same.) First, they could put on a fat suit so they are of similar weight to a typical patient. Use me for an example. My 14-year-old weighs what I've lost. There is no way that I could now pick him up and carry him around all day, especially on my stomach.

Live my former life for a few months. Take the five+ medications that the typical patient is on; try to ride on a plane, shop at the mall, carry in the groceries, go to a job interview, go to the movies, or park and shop at Wal-Mart. Then start the surgical weight loss process. Come to a two-hour seminar. Help me fill out the eight-page questionnaire; request my medical records for the last five years from my primary care physician and specialists. Go with me to see my primary care physician to discuss surgery and to request their approval for surgery.

Join me for my psychological evaluation; have your blood drawn with me; come to my three-hour class to get ready for surgery. Sit with me at my house for the anywhere from two to eight weeks it can take to hear from the insurance company if I'm approved (and, please, cry with me when I'm denied). Drink the mag citrate with me. (Okay, you don't have to follow me into the bathroom, but do stay close outside.) Then come follow me through surgery. Be in the room with me four hours after surgery when I get up to walk for the first time.

Get the idea? Yeah, right: it was a walk in the park.

It *is* major surgery, and it can cost you your life, not to mention your life savings and untold complications. How is that ever the easy way out? Who

would ever choose this route, unless they had exhausted all hope of any other alternatives?

Was it a hard decision to have surgery? Yes. Did I research it a lot? Yes. Would I do it again? Yes. I would have it once a month if that is what it would take to keep the weight off. Was I worried about dying? Yes. I've read that the mortality rate for this surgery is somewhere between 0.5% (1:200) to 2% (2:100).

The bottom line is that it's an individual decision. Discuss it with friends and family, but ultimately, each person much decide for him or herself.

I now have multiple blessings—I'm at my ideal weight; I love my family, friends, and life; and I have the job of my dreams. I've been hired as surgical weight loss coordinator at the medical center in my town, and I'm striving to develop the finest WLS clinic in the world. I often think back to the days when I used to be greeted, "Good morning, Chub-Chub." Now I get to greet and welcome other chub-chubs to the *losing side* after their weight loss surgery. What a wonderful world I live in, and how far I've come!

6

A Friend Indeed for a Friend in Need

by
Ken McLaughlin

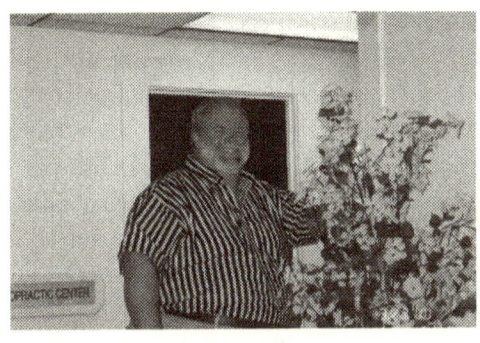

Sometimes it takes an intervention to make important things happen. I don't mean the kind of intervention that results in a midnight kidnapping and that might be arranged by family or friends for someone who has a substance abuse problem. The kind of intervention I am referring to is one where someone who deeply cares about you steps in and confronts you with the harsh realities about your obesity because they want you to live.

It takes a special kind of courage to speak truth to someone who doesn't want to hear it. Sure, I've been told that I was courageous to choose to have my gastric bypass surgery but, in my opinion, that wasn't the real element of courage in the process that finally resulted in me doing something about my morbid obesity. The real courage was in my friend being brave enough to intervene and confront me about my deteriorating health and my future (or lack thereof) if I stayed at the weight that was slowly, but surely, killing me.

Because Brian cared enough to penetrate my denial with his sincere desire to keep me alive, I ultimately chose to have gastric bypass surgery. As a result, I feel like I have been given back my life. In February of 2003, he sat me down and expressed his concerns for my health. In addition to pointing out the fact that at my current weight I wasn't likely to live many more years, he said something else that really got to me. He said, "You're just not fun to do things with anymore."

Those words did get to me. I understood what he meant. I couldn't walk *any* distance without stopping to rest. When I went to hockey games with him I hung over into his seat so I knew that I wasn't much fun to sit next to. In fact, many times I would look around for two empty seats so that I could sit by myself without cramping Brian or anyone else. I was *always* tired from the exertion of moving my 450-pound body. A few months before our talk, Brian and I had gone to the Breeders Cup race at Santa Anita and, when we were walking to and from the grandstand to the parking lot, I would have to stop every fifty yards or so to catch my breath.

But I also sensed how difficult it was for Brian to talk to me about this subject. It had to be because he was also worried about our friendship. As Brian later told me, if he had not talked with me about my weight and then something happened to me, he would have had a hard time living with that. I had to respect what our friendship meant to him and to take his words seriously. To not listen—really listen—would have been to disrespect my friend and our friendship.

So I began to explore my options. I had been through every possible diet and weight loss program, so I needed to find reliable information about more drastic, more permanent solutions. I had heard about gastric bypass surgery, but when I had previously looked into it I found out that my health insurance would not pay for it. The first bit of good news I learned in my new research was that many insurance companies were now paying for weight loss surgery. That removed a big obstacle, particularly for my wife, who already opposed any consideration of such an extreme and drastic surgical procedure.

Since weight loss surgery was now an affordable possibility, I started to explore my local options, trying to identify doctors and hospitals that specialized in bariatric surgery. This turned out to be more of a challenge than I thought it would. I live in the San Francisco Bay Area and assumed that there must be many qualified doctors who performed this kind of medical procedure. While I could find some doctors and hospitals, the greater problem was finding a qualified, *experienced* surgeon who was also included in my PPO health insurance plan.

In the process of all my searching, I joined a bariatric support group. It was there that I learned about what Kaiser Permanente was doing in conjunction with Pacific Bariatric in San Diego. In earlier research, I had learned about Pacific Bariatric and their leadership in bariatric medicine. The more I learned from the members of my support group, the more excited I became about the possibility of changing my life. And the more certain I became that Pacific Bariatric was the right clinic to trust with my body and my life.

As I was learning more about weight loss surgery, including the risks and after-effects, it didn't seem as if I had any other viable or realistic options. In seeing the postoperative members of my support group, I could—for the first time ever—see the prospect of a future that would allow me to enjoy life again, albeit with food being much less important in my life than it had always been.

If I didn't choose surgery, it seemed likely that my body would continue to break down under the merciless burden of its own weight. I would spend less time with my friend, and I would most likely die an early death due to my obesity. Weight loss surgery could give me the chance to walk pain free, play golf, travel by air, and generally improve the quality of my life.

Ironically, my wife and I had been thinking of switching our health plan to the Kaiser HMO when it came time for open enrollment. It seemed as if things were starting to fall into place for me, even though my wife was still not in favor of my having surgery.

Cheryl had several very serious reservations about my having the surgery. First, she was genuinely concerned about the risky nature of the procedure. At the Pacific Bariatric orientation we attended, the surgeon (Dr. Leo Murphy, who wound up being my surgeon) pointed out that as elective surgeries go, this one is very risky—like any major surgery for a person with comorbid (life-threatening) conditions. (The general rate of fatalities from weight loss surgery is at least 1 in 200, or 0.05%) He said that on a scale of 1 to 10, with 10 being an organ transplant, gastric bypass is a 9. He may have been saying that to get people's attention, and he certainly got my wife's.

Cheryl is also one of those people who feel that weight loss surgery is taking "the easy way out." Many times she has told me that she didn't think I had tried hard enough or used enough will power to lose whatever weight I needed to lose. We talked about how important food had become in our lives, as she enjoys cooking and I enjoy eating her cooking. She felt that if I had this surgery there would be little for us to do together.

I tried to use her very own argument as a way of showing her that I truly needed to do something drastic about my weight if we were going to enjoy very many more years together. The fact of the matter was that at my present weight and in my present condition, eating was about all we had to enjoy together. We couldn't do any travel that involved flying anywhere and our sex life had become nonexistent.

I am sure that there were also issues involving her own insecurities if I suddenly lost massive amounts of weight and transformed my appearance, but we never really discussed them. To be fair, though, her daughter is also considering weight loss surgery and Cheryl is not in favor of Julie doing it either—even now that she has seen for herself the positive results of my surgery, and the fact that we are now able to plan some long-anticipated trips, and that she's found some recipes that allow her to cook well and still satisfy my special needs as a WLS post-op person.

In July of 2003 I was able to switch to Kaiser. Leading up to that time I had gotten lots of information from other Kaiser patients as to how to proceed once I switched. My first course of action was to request a primary care physician who had experience with getting a patient through the approval process. That has proved to be some of the best advice I got from my support group.

My new doctor immediately recognized me as a good candidate for weight loss surgery and started requesting the tests he knew I would need in order to get an approval from Kaiser for my surgery. As I guess with most bariatric protocols, there was a significant gauntlet of interviews and tests that I had to complete in order to get approved for weight loss surgery by Kaiser. Much of the process deals with your weight and weight-loss history.

For me, my first experience with having weight gain problems occurred in my mid-twenties. At that time, however, I was able to lose the extra pounds through diet control and successfully kept the weight off for several years. However, my problem with weight manifested itself again about ten years later. I went through the usual attempts to control my eating, including the early version of the Atkins diet, fen-phen, Weight Watchers, hypnosis, and so on—I tried them all. I was certainly motivated to keep the weight off because I refereed college basketball games, but knew that I would be dropped if I couldn't control my weight. The best I ever did was to lose just under fifty pounds. What I regained was always more than what I had lost.

When I did receive my WLS approval, it wasn't to go to Pacific Bariatric in San Diego, but to Kaiser's new facility in South San Francisco. Through my support group I had become very familiar with how Pacific Bariatric did things and that was where I wanted my surgery. Once again, my primary physician was supportive of me and made his own request that I be assigned to Pacific Bariatric.

Now there was another round of tests, measurements, and hopes for approval. The first step was to attend an orientation meeting. As Dr. Murphy talked about the risks, he also talked about the successes. I learned that the procedure I would undergo was the Roux-en-Y gastric bypass. A recent patient also spoke and shared her experience with the audience. It was hard not to get excited about the possibility of getting back some form of a normal life. I was committed to doing whatever I needed to do in order to be approved by Pacific Bariatric for my surgery.

Their big emphasis was on presurgical weight loss and physical conditioning. My official weigh-in was at 451 pounds. The rule of thumb was that I should expect to lose about 10% of that weight *before* I could have my surgery. On December 1, I joined a health club and found a personal trainer. I also started to replace one meal a day with a protein shake. The other great piece of advice I got from my support group was to put together a diary and portfolio of my training sessions and my daily menu. That way, when I met with my surgeon from PB he would be able to see that I was serious about being successful.

During all this time I did not share my intentions with very many people, including my brothers and sister. Brian, of course, knew, as did a select few of my closest friends. I was still so afraid of failure that I didn't want to broadcast my desperation to the world prematurely. However, their support was absolutely critical to keeping my motivation. Between them and the support group I was able to stay focused on what I needed to do. When I realized that I wasn't losing the weight I needed to, my support group suggested that I replace two meals a day with the protein shakes.

Having a strong support system has proven to be one of the most important elements of both my presurgical success and my postsurgical progress. As I mentioned, I told only a few close friends, and did not tell my other family members or the members of my Rotary Club. Fear of failing once again is tough to overcome. Where I did find support was from staff at the health club and from other members who saw me at the club on a daily basis. I was open and honest with them about my plans and surgical intentions.

To my surprise and delight, I got lots of encouragement from people I didn't even know very well. Maybe they had previously dealt with their own weight issues and had some sense of what I was trying to confront. The positive environment at the gym made it much, much easier to go, even on days when I was tired and would have preferred to go home and park my butt in front of the television. Between the people at the health club, my bariatric support group, and my closest friends, I was able to overcome the negativity that still existed at home. The support made me feel that I really could achieve my objective.

At the point that I eventually told my siblings and the members of my Rotary Club, I got overwhelming support and I felt a bit foolish for having worried about their reactions. In retrospect, while I realize that such a surgery is a personal matter and one that I felt embarrassed about, I think that being up front about it can garner much more positive support than criticism and is thus well worth the risk.

Just seven and a half weeks after beginning my diet and exercise program, it was time to see if I had hit my target weight in order to get my surgery scheduled. When it was my turn to step on the scale, I emptied my pockets, took off my shoes, and held my breath to see what number appeared. I made it with four pounds to spare. Now, my objective was to not go backward.

My surgical date was set for Monday, March 1. I would go down to San Diego on Friday to have my pre-op meeting and final weigh-in. Leading up to that date, I continued with my water aerobics and pushed myself in the gym. Upon arriving at Scripps Hospital in San Diego for my pre-op meeting, I discovered I was the only man in the group of people who would be having their surgery on Monday. As we were called, one at a time, to get weighed, most of the women were very nervous about whether they had gained weight and might risk having their surgery cancelled. Each of them came in under their required weight, anywhere from two to eight pounds. When it was announced that I was thirty-seven pounds under target, there were a lot of oohs and ahs from the rest of the group. That really made me feel good about all my hard work.

One of the most positive things I did while still obese was to find self-acceptance in who I was, as a person, regardless of my weight, in order to avoid feeling the same sense of shame that so many overweight people do.

My wife was still very much opposed to my having the surgery. She feared that our life together, as we currently enjoyed it, would come to an end. I tried to explain to her that too much of that life revolved around food, and that for the health of both of us, it could not continue. Saturday night would be my final meal as the "fat Ken". For my wife's sake, I wanted it to be special. I made reservations at a restaurant that overlooked the ocean and we were seated where we could watch the sunset while dining. The food was as special as I hoped it would be, and my last big meal was lobster Thermidor.

My surgery was scheduled for 1:30 in the afternoon, so I had to be at the hospital about mid-morning. I think that the waiting was the hardest part of the entire experience. Eventually, it was time to get onto the gurney and be rolled into the depths of the hospital, where the operating rooms were. I saw my surgeon, met my anesthesiologist, and that was about the last thing I remembered until I saw my wife back in my room after surgery. I was still groggy and could only briefly acknowledge her presence and then drifted back to sleep.

At 10 PM I finally came out of my sleep altogether, and it was time for me to take my first steps. I was in a special bed that could be tilted up so that I could literally walk out of the bed standing up. With my IV bottle and stand on one hand and the nurse on the other, I began my walk around the hospital floor. No pain! What a surprise and relief! I also felt surprisingly strong. When we completed one circuit of the floor, my nurse asked if I was ready to go back to my room. I told her no, that I wanted to go around again. I still felt no pain and while I did feel a bit tired from the additional exertion, I had a real sense of confidence that things were going well.

I guess I really knew that I was starting to recover quickly as I realized how uncomfortable the urinary catheter was and I made enough of a fuss that they removed it about 5 AM Tuesday morning. That, of course, forced me to have to get up to use the bathroom, but it also encouraged me to get out and walk more often. Still, I wasn't feeling any pain from my surgery. At 11 AM, the WLS patients were to assemble in a room for a session of light exercise. I saw the ladies whom I had met at our meeting on Friday as well as some of the patients from previous days. Most of the others from my group did not seem to be doing as well as I felt I was doing, and a couple of them went back to their rooms before the session was over.

Under the arrangement that Kaiser had with Pacific Bariatric, I would be staying in San Diego until the following Monday, when I would have my final checkup and then, hopefully, be released to go home. My wife was going to return home the day after my surgery, so she stopped by the hospital before heading for the airport. She told me that after my operation, my surgeon, Dr. Leo Murphy, came out and told her that he could really tell the benefits of my presurgical weight loss and physical conditioning. He explained to her that he had plenty of extra skin to work with when stitching me back up and that my muscle tone was excellent. I was already anxious to get out of the hospital and back to the hotel.

Wednesday morning Dr. Murphy was in to see me early and decided that there was no need for me to stay in until Thursday. I could check out later that morning but, meanwhile, could get out of my hospital gown and back into regular clothes. I was all dressed when it was time for that morning's exercise class and it was fun to go down there knowing I would be released soon. The others from my group looked better than they had the day before, but still seemed to be suffering more than they would have liked.

In the days that I was on my own at the hotel, the hours I spent on the treadmill back at my gym were paying off. As much as I am not a big fan of just walking, I was able to get out and walk up and down the street to get my exercise and some sunshine. What was kind of fun at the hotel was that there develops an instant sense of community among the bariatric patients, and we became supportive of each other. We would ask each other who our surgeon was and talk about good places to go walking away from the hospital neighborhood.

My visit to San Diego ended on schedule on Monday when Dr. Murphy released me to go back home. In just that first week I managed to lose ten pounds and I was amazed at how fast my excess weight was falling off. As I sat on the airplane for my return to San Jose, I had the optimistic thought that this would be the last flight where I would have to ask the attendant for a seat belt extender.

Two months after my surgery, I was down a total of 120 lbs. I had lost fifty before surgery and seventy since March 1. I had been back in the gym getting back into shape and now felt I was ready to play my first round of golf since my surgery. My plan was to go up to Lake Tahoe for that round of golf. Unfortunately, the success of my weight loss created an unanticipated side effect that had nearly tragic consequences.

As with many obese people, I was on blood pressure medication. Thirty days after my surgery I met with my primary care physician and, at the time, there was no indication that an adjustment needed to be made in the dosage of my medication. In driving to Lake Tahoe, the top is Echo Summit at an elevation of 7800 feet before starting the descent. Once starting down, heading toward the lake, the road is narrow and winding. Within just 100 yards after starting that descent, I suddenly felt very dizzy and could not keep my car between the lines on the road. I knew that I didn't want to cross over the center line and risk hitting another car coming up the mountain. To the right of me, however, was a short wall and a 1,000-foot drop.

Before getting dizzy I had down-shifted my car into third gear so that my engine would help keep me from going too fast, so I was probably going only 25–30 miles per hour. Still, I couldn't keep control of the car and hit up against the right wall. At that point the world was really spinning around and I knew I was drifting to my left across the center line. I remember thinking, please don't let me hit anyone else. Luck was on my side that morning as no other car was coming, and I crashed my car into the granite boulders on the mountain side of the highway.

While not actually injured from the crash, I was not feeling very well because I had been hit by the car's airbags and was sore from the seat belt and shoulder harness. My car was equipped with OnStar and they contacted emergency personnel, who ultimately had to cut me out of my car before loading me into the ambulance. After about four hours in the emergency room, I was told I could be released as there didn't seem to be anything seriously wrong with me. I did notice, however, that my blood pressure seemed unusually low.

When I was able to return to San Jose and meet with my primary care physician, he had me go through a series of exams including wearing a heart monitor for twenty-four hours to see if there was anything there that could have been the cause of my dizziness. Meanwhile, he took me completely off my blood pressure medication. When all was said and done, my doctor concluded that my 120-pound weight loss, the full dosage of medication, and the high elevation, which will cause blood pressure to lower, all came together at the wrong time and resulted in my becoming dizzy and losing control of my car.

I recently had my six-month checkup. Both my surgeon and I were amazed at my progress. I had lost 184 pounds from my beginning weight taken at my orientation some ten months earlier. Even more important than the weight loss were the other physiological changes in my body. Since the last set of body measurements taken eight months ago, I had lost two-thirds of all my body fat weight and had reduced my body fat percentage from 38.6% down to 21.2%. Given that I have the usual apron hanging down from my belly that weighs 15–20 pounds and will have to be dealt with surgically, I really felt on top of the world.

Along with the pounds of fat, my sleep apnea had disappeared, and I was able to stop sleeping with my CPAP machine. As hard as I thought it might be to learn how to sleep and breathe without it, my greatest difficulty was learning to sleep without the gentle noise of the machine. It was too quiet at night. Being able to sleep without the CPAP machine probably rates as my single biggest "wow, I can do that" moment since my surgery. Getting off that machine was a dream come true.

Being able to play golf again, and to be pain free, also ranks right up there in my list of most special moments. Being able to bend over and tie my shoes or trim my toenails may not seem like a big deal, but, since I haven't been able to do those simple tasks for years, that's significant. In a couple of months I am looking forward to flying without a seatbelt extender and being able to comfortably use the airplane bathroom.

With every new thing I can do, I give a quiet word of thanks to my friend Brian. Without his caring and courageous confrontation, I might never have gotten to enjoy my second chance at living a long, healthy, and mobile life.

Throughout this process I have attempted to go back and figure out how I got into this situation in the first place. I have yet to understand what my issues are with food beyond the fact that *eating makes me feel good*. The further I go along, the more I realize that my real challenges probably lie ahead of me. I have learned that I do not suffer from dumping when I eat something with sugar or too much fat. That is a good news/bad news situation.

It will mean that I will have to be ever vigilant in regards to not slipping back into bad habits, particularly when it comes to snacking. That is why the bariatric support group will continue to have an important role in my life, as those will be people who will identify with many of my issues and help remind me of what I need to do to not regain weight.

It cannot be stressed enough that surgery is not for everyone.

My youngest brother, who is also morbidly obese, hasn't reached that point yet where he feels surgery is appropriate for him. He may, however, change his mind once he sees me at his fiftieth birthday celebration. As with anyone considering such a course of action, I advised him to visit a bariatric support group and to research the Internet for information.

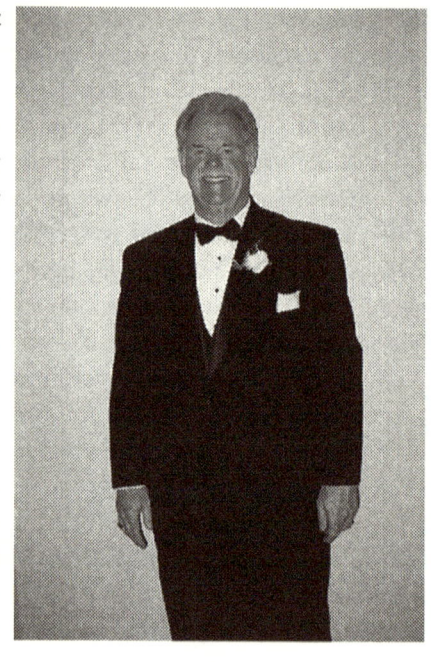

Surgery was the right choice for me. By losing my excess weight, I have significantly diminished my mortality risk factors. My blood pressure is normal, and I am no longer on medication. My sleep apnea has disappeared. At the last test, my cholesterol was at 138 and my triglycerides were 59. Short of stepping off the curb and getting hit by a bus, I've got every reason to believe that I can live a long, healthy, and active life. All because my friend Brian showed great courage and intervened in my life. What a positive difference a loving, caring, and committed friend can make!

7

Less of Me
Is More

by
Hillary Bowden

I think I may have been thin twice as an adult—both times for about fifteen minutes!

I was raised in a middle-class, white, Christian home, but with a mother who had latent tendencies toward "Jewish mama syndrome"—the condition that leads one to feed those they love in order to show and prove their love.

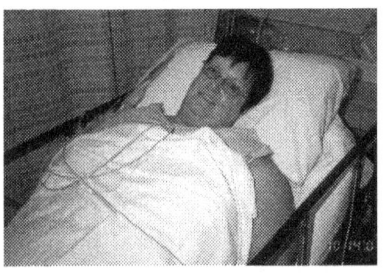

I was almost ten pounds at birth—a portent of things to come? My first memory of being tormented about my weight was in the fifth grade. I had started my menstrual cycle the summer after fourth grade, and the boys noticed my early developing bosom. Well, they delighted in shoving oranges up their shirts and making fun of me. I can, to this day, remember my poor male teacher having to drag me out of the girls' bathroom where I had taken up residence and sought sanctuary.

My first diet began shortly after that. I can recall eating hard-boiled eggs and toast and not much else! My mother was using Ayds candies as a diet aid, so I tried those as well.

I never met a *dry* noodle or piece of toast. My mom had taken chef's classes on the East Coast in the forties—back in the days when real, calorie-laden, honest-to-goodness butter reigned supreme and sauces demanded lots of it! We ate lobster Newburg, lobster Thermidor, eggs Benedict, wonderfully rich biscuits dripping with butter and honey, and so much more.

A special treat I remember was that night out where I met my true love: the French pastry cart. I was instantly smitten. Just the sight of the cart at another diner's table would set my poor childish chin aquiver...would I be allowed to choose between an éclair or a Napoleon? Or would my dad be in a dour mood and decide we'd skip dessert tonight? Oh, the horror of it all! A tryst missed.

And so it began. We lived in a rural area without other children nearby so I developed skills that didn't require playmates: a passion for reading and playing alone in the fields with just the company of my dog. I loved being around the adults who worked for my folks in the family business. They ate well and loved to share their lunches. Some had strange exotic fare, like borscht (with sour cream); others had plain, hardy meals, including rich desserts (again with the chocolate!). Although I was a pudgy kid, I was pretty active. When I began school, I was quite the tomboy and could really throw a baseball far—which won the hearts of most of the little boys and turned the frilly little girls against me. That was just fine with me!

When I started to mature, and curves replaced rolls of baby fat, I discovered that those little boys liked the curves even more than the baseballs I used to throw! Unfortunately, all that attention led to an early marriage, a baby, and yes—a weight gain of sixty pounds. That shot me up to 180. I lost some weight but then became pregnant again, and yet again. It was the old story of easy on, hell to get off!

The first diet I tried was after the birth of my first child: starvation. I soon graduated to injections of urine from pregnant women; Weight Watchers (back in the day when you *had* to eat so many ounces of liver per week!); hypnosis; NutriSystem; Jenny Craig, more injections of vitamins; low-fat, low-carb, soup diets, fruit diets; Atkins, Metrical; liquid protein; and these are just the diets that come to mind! Every new fad that came down the pike, I'd try. Sadly, I always failed. The diets didn't fail—I did.

I managed to lose enough on a starvation diet to go to Hawaii in 1989. I was determined to be able to wear shorts for the first time in years. Although I looked okay (at 140 pounds), my insecurity wouldn't let me wear a swimsuit. At forty-two years of age, I was still hung up on the "perfect body" concept. "Unless you look like a model, you don't wear a swimsuit in public." And I wished everyone knew that. I'd look at obese women in swimsuits and be appalled. I was *so judgmental*. About them. About myself.

This is the first time that I had actually used exercise as a tool, along with dieting. I used several videotapes, alternating them so that I had cardio, stretching, walking, etc. I felt more youthful than I had in ages. I stood taller, held myself with a more self-confident carriage, and my back didn't ache nearly as much. We walked all over Oahu and I lost four pounds that week. My exercise had revved up my metabolism to a higher level that allowed me to eat more than usual and actually lose weight! Wow! That was a new concept! Why then, did I stop? I fell back into old habits and relapsed into laziness once again. Once again, I failed.

Even at my largest (265 pounds), I only allowed myself to look like a matron in public. "No upper arms revealed; no thighs bared. Keep the children away! Don't let the sight of a fat lady scare the little ones!"

Shame was my most powerful and destructive demon of all. I was so ashamed of what I'd become. I totally lost myself, my personage, if you will, inside of the fatness.

Besides that joyful trip to Hawaii, the only other time I was thin was after my thirty-year-old husband died in an auto accident less than a mile from our home. I was left with three children under age twelve. Grief ate away at me, quite literally, until I regained my former lean frame. I couldn't lose the weight for my husband while he was alive, but after his death, the weight came off. Another failure, more shame.

I stayed at 130 pounds until I remarried. This time it wasn't birthing babies that caused my weight to climb again, but complacency. I had married a wonderful, committed man, and I knew that he wouldn't leave me if I plumped up a bit. True to his word, he didn't, but our marriage suffered, as I continued to suffer from the indignity of my lost self-esteem. After all, he didn't marry a 265-pound woman! That wasn't in the contract.

My blessed mother found out that she had cancer, and within three weeks she was dead. During that period, she begged me to lose weight and not let it ruin the rest of my life the same way that her obesity had impacted hers.

Ten years later, I made the decision to have gastric bypass surgery. All the pleading, the tears, the fighting over my weight by all the people who loved me couldn't persuade me to take control of my body, my life, and my weight issue. Then one day, my inner lightbulb suddenly lit up. I realized that the rest of my life was *now*. How many more days, months, and years did I have left? Did I want to spend it with gimpy knees that would give out and leave me lying on the ground, with acid reflux and high blood pressure, with depression and sleepless nights? My answer was a resounding no!

I began to read about this barbaric procedure called *stomach stapling*. There were so many side effects: chronic diarrhea, vomiting, nausea, and even the possibility of death. I had taken risks with my health but this was going too far! But as advances were made and the procedures were refined and perfected, I started noticing advertisements in our local newspaper for seminars promoting "gastric bypass." Right! Surgeons harvesting new fields from which to fill their coffers; that was really going to make me change my bias in thinking. But then curiosity got the better of me. I had friends who were actually undergoing this radical procedure *and* were losing weight! I decided to attend one of these phony-baloney seminars and sit back and scoff.

As my husband and I entered the seminar, I noticed that the majority of the attendees were markedly obese. Some were in wheelchairs; others on "scooters." They had an air of hopelessness about them. I thought to myself, "Is that what it's going to take before I do something about my weight? Let myself get so large I won't be able to walk?" The thought paralyzed me emotionally. As the two surgeons began to speak, I slowly noticed a light starting to shine behind eyes that had been dimmed of hope.

The physicians were not offering a magic bullet but a life-saving tool! One that—if used properly—could help all of us become victors instead of victims.

It took another year of further study and evaluation of the process before I decided to have the surgery. I am extremely fortunate that I work for a government agency so that my health benefits are excellent and paid for the surgery. I was only off work for two weeks (mainly because of a co-worker who was very unkind and highly critical of weight loss surgery). I was determined to show her that even after an open Roux-en-Y gastric bypass surgery, I would tough it out and show up for work. I did!

The night before my surgery, I was no more nervous than anyone else would have been undergoing any other major surgery. I was just anxious to get it over with and to get on with the business of living. I was more afraid of failing to be a success than I ever was of dying. I realized the risks of any surgery, but the cloud that hung over my future far outweighed the risks.

At the time of surgery I was on twelve medications, including prescriptions for high blood pressure, acid reflux, irritable bowel syndrome, anxiety and depression, and the pain from my arthritic knees. Now, I take only five medications! Most of my meds were discontinued immediately after surgery, to my surprise, relief, and great joy.

My surgeon was outstanding! I couldn't have asked for a better one. Part of the process I went through in the year before I decided to opt for the surgery was to check out the surgeons (and their mortality rates) at the hospitals. The range of rates of death (0.5–1%) or complications (5–10%) from weight loss surgery are comparable to those for most other major surgeries. One of the reasons that the procedure can be "high risk" is that so many morbidly obese patients suffer comorbidities, such as chronic kidney failure, chronic heart disease, diabetes, and other life-threatening conditions.

Many people—family, friends, and co-workers—have heard horror stories about someone who knows someone, or who has a cousin who has a friend who…. So out of their concern for my well-being, some tried to persuade me not to have the surgery. And, of course, there were others who live under a constant cloud of doom and gloom who tried to convince me to stay the same as I was, because being thin was perceived as a threat or competition.

My husband and children were extremely cooperative and cheered me on. My family is my richest blessing. My youngest daughter is thirty-four and has stayed slim—even after two children. My oldest daughter is thirty-nine and fights the good fight to stay thin. My son is getting a bit of a "spare tire" around his middle but, fortunately, none of them show any signs of becoming morbidly obese and following in my footsteps.

As we drove home from the hospital, my husband needed to eat. We were at a nice café and he was so hesitant to eat in front of me. I kept reassuring him that it was fine, and that we had to start the process somewhere, sometime. He did a lot of apologizing at first, but eventually he got used to eating in front of me. I was one month out of surgery when Thanksgiving rolled around. I had one little tiny taste of everything—it really didn't bother me. I focused on my protein intake and had a wonderful visit with my family. Honestly, they felt much worse about my eating limitations than I did. It was hard to convince them that I didn't feel as if I was being punished. I truly wasn't hungry and did not feel deprived in the least.

I never dreamt I could go six months without a diet cola or a steak. I did! I followed my surgeon's rules to the ultimate degree. I still have a protein shake every morning, but I mix it up with fruit and instant coffee. I've gone back to diet cola, which I need to curtail. I can eat anything I want except rice—especially the rice from Chinese restaurants. I do not drink alcohol because even a sip of a cocktail sends me reeling!

Along with the feelings of shame I felt as an obese youth and then an obese woman, I have dealt with and am still dealing with my fear of failure. I am an emotional eater. I "eat" my anger because I have never found an acceptable outlet for expressing and releasing it.

As a child, I received a sound spanking for throwing rocks in a field because I was mad about some perceived injustice. As a young wife, when I once became angry with my husband, he disappeared for a weekend. I soon learned that exhibiting any outward sign of anger was not going to yield positive results. So I ate, and gorged myself at the feast festering inside.

Today, my intellect helps me understand that this is destructive behavior and that some physical exercise, or attacking my anger in a direct and positive way, will not only help me deal with my anger, but will also enhance and enrich the way I live my life. My challenge is to undo all those years of listening to the wrong messages. My job is to learn how to listen to my body's hunger and to only eat when I'm *truly* hungry.

I have recently undergone another traumatic emotional loss. My first reaction was to overeat. I quickly regained five of those pounds I had fought so hard to lose. The old messages started playing over and over again in my brain: "See? You went through all the surgery and for what? You're still going to fail! You're going to wind up fat again." I must stay eternally vigilant!

I have come to understand, finally, that emotional trauma can be healthy! The dark night of the soul gives us sustenance, but not for our physical being. It is only through the trials of this life that we are able to grow as humans and become able to reach out and offer comfort and solace to others who are hurting. I am working through the depression, anger, hurt, loss, and grief—but this time, I put my fork down.

This journey to and from my weight loss surgery has gifted me with one epiphany after another. I have forgiven myself for being human. I have allowed myself to be who I was created to be: shaped by my creator and given certain talents, skills, and abilities. I have mellowed—some just from the process of aging, but also, and mostly, from the process of becoming thin and learning, once again, to love myself. Today I look in wonder at the photos of who I was, and I remember all the pain, the shame, the guilt, the hiding, the secrecy. And now it's okay.

I kept a journal religiously. Last night I reread through some of the entries as I started down the road of discovery and recovery. Incredibly, I lost thirty-five pounds the first month!

I forgot how difficult it was to eat chicken at first. It almost always made me vomit. I spent thirty precious minutes of a Moody Blues concert in the bathroom, trying to convince the small piece of chicken I had eaten for dinner to remove itself from my newly created and tiny stomach pouch.

I had several episodes of dumping, usually due to eating too quickly. The worst episode I endured was trying to eat white rice from a Chinese restaurant—the sticky kind of rice. When I got back to the office after lunch, I actually thought I was having a heart attack. The pain centered in the middle of my chest and was so intense I truly thought, "This is it." I made it to the restroom just in the nick of time!

Not to be gross, but I found it very interesting that the vomit at first is nothing but foam! The first time I threw up, I hurt so bad that I expected a clump of food to erupt from my gut, not foam! It's all so very different from presurgical up-chucking.

Another of my strange reactions is to sugar. The first time I tried to eat a little ice cream, I almost fell asleep in mid-taste. The sugar just instantly hit my system and my blood sugars went haywire. Then I broke out in a sweat. Once I figured all this out, and understood what my body was telling me, I became more and more comfortable with the whole process.

Another weird thing my body now does to alert me to slow down is that I start to sneeze! When I'm eating anything fast and not paying attention, I'll start sneezing. It's as if my stomach is trying to make room.

I have not used the tool of exercise since my surgery as I should have, especially for a woman of my age. Consequently, I now have to worry about the infamous dowager's hump. I can tell that I have lost massive amounts of muscle and have become very bony. My knees are knobby and my collarbones look like bicycle handlebars! My parrot, who loves to sit on my shoulder, thinks I have new perches built in, just for him!

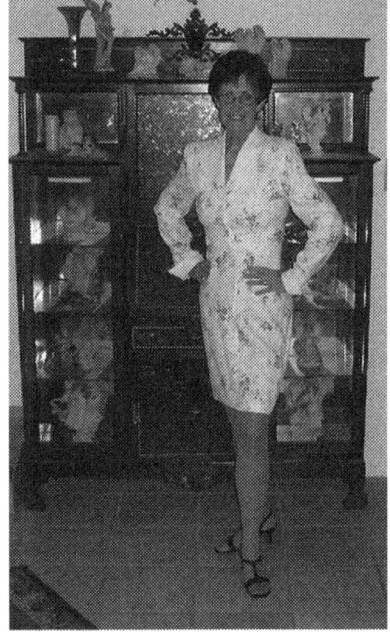

It really is imperative—and so very helpful and energy-effective—to get up and move: walk, stretch, leap for joy! I have dusted off my "Strong Women Live Longer" videotape, along with some others, and am determined to walk tall and stand proudly once again.

I have heard so many people say that, despite all the difficult challenges, downsides, and tradeoffs, they would have the surgery all over again. Count me in as one of those people. Sure, I may look like a shar-pei without my clothes on but that's okay. We went to Kauai, Hawaii, this spring. I wore a swimsuit and didn't give a hoot about my crinkly thighs!

My bottom line: my pre-op weight was 261; today I weigh 135. My waist has shrunk from 47 1/2 to 29 inches; my bust has reduced from 53 to 36; I've lost 5 inches of flab from my upper arms, 16 inches off my hips, and a full foot off my thighs. I've transformed from a size 22–24 to a size 4–6, and my underwear look like they belong to some skinny kid.

I've gotten my body and my life back. And less of me is *so much more*!

8

WLS Saved This Farm Boy's Life!

by
Jeffery McCreary

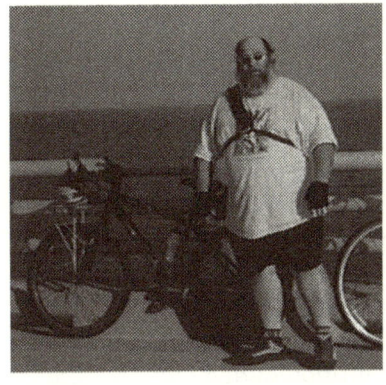

I was the husky one in our farm family, but I always felt like I belonged. My mother and grandfather both weighed 385 pounds, and my great-grandfather exceeded the 400-pound mark. So I always felt a special kinship within my family—I was just another hefty chip off the old block—and my size was nothing special or unusual. Although I carried a lot of weight, I was still one of the smallest and scrawniest members of my family, so naturally they called me "small fry."

I was born a fat baby, and I stayed fat and chubby. In our family, with our genes, if you weren't overweight, there was definitely something wrong with you! (My father, who stood 5'3" and weighed 125 pounds dripping wet, was the one glaring exception.) By third grade, I was well into the 176-pound range and headed ever upward and onward.

I was used to the hard work required on a working farm. Baling hay, cleaning out stalls, hauling 50- and 100-pound feed bags—all this felt like child's play to me. In my world on the farm, people were judged not by what they weighed, but by how much they could lift and how much work they could do. I could lift massive loads, and I could work my heart out. My size was one of my greatest assets—at least at this early stage in my life.

I rode my bicycle everywhere. I swam in the bayous. I hiked the levees, went fishing, ran the fields, and climbed the trees. I played high school football, and even joined the baseball and tennis teams. I was always active, and my 300+ pounds never seemed to slow me down. My football coaches felt my size was a real advantage on the field, and when baseball season rolled around, I wasn't concerned about running, because I was so strong. When I connected with a pitch, my strength usually resulted in a homerun.

Growing up on a farm, there was always an abundance of food, and all food was comfort food. I remember the farm table piled high with biscuits and gravy, mashed taters, and fried chicken. Not to mention gumbo; corn bread; macaroni and cheese; cakes, pies, and cookies; and homemade juices and wines. Fresh-grown produce, the bounty of our fields, was always on our table. We grew nearly everything we ate. And what we didn't grow, we traded with our relatives for what they had readily available, including rice, fresh seafood, beef, pork, and wild game.

I always had a good appetite, but in my family, when momma filled your plate, you'd better eat it all! Looking back, it was a fairly well-balanced menu, including vegetables, proteins, fruits, breads, and dairy, but what I remember most, in retrospect, was how much food was always stacked on my plate. I never blamed my mom for making me the fat kid. We were *all* fat (except for my skinny dad)!

When I joined the U.S. Navy, the recruiter was certain that boot camp would "slim me down," but that never quite happened. I marched, paraded, and drilled, but I just became stronger and somewhat leaner—never much lighter, much to the Navy's chagrin. The military seemed determined to get me down to their ideal weight, which they very nearly did. An extended stay in the local military hospital to recover from dehydration and malnutrition during my time in boot camp was the only result of their fixation.

Seven years later the Navy discovered this wonderful new liquid protein diet, and once again it was "suggested" that I try this in another attempt to reduce my excess weight. I was pleasantly surprised to find myself losing weight, but found it difficult to maintain a working relationship with my squadron because of the restrictions (and complications) of a purely liquid protein meal replacement regimen. Finally, one morning, I was awoken by severe pain and cramping. I fell to the floor and was unable to get back up. After being rushed to the base hospital, the squadron flight surgeon took me off the experimental diet and put me back on regular Navy chow. The pounds lost returned with a vengeance (and compounded interest), but I was able to regain my strength, and rigorous weight training soon enabled me to return to work.

After leaving the Navy, I found steady employment with a municipality in Virginia, and even though I was healthy enough to pass the physical, I was unsatisfied with the direction my weight was taking. I was leading a fairly active lifestyle at 300+ pounds, but for every 10–20 pounds I would lose on a diet, 30–40 pounds would soon take their place.

We were an active family—camping, bicycling, hiking, and such. Whole wheat bread was the norm, with plenty of vegetables, and staying away from the cakes and pies and other such sugary desserts. My food treats were fruit (not sugar) based, but I still did not seem to lose any weight. Since my sixteenth birthday, I had consistently maintained an average weight of 350 pounds. As a young boy on a farm, that was okay, and I maintained my strength and fitness through long hours in the field and working with the animals. But at age fifty-three, living in the city and having a municipal job, I just could not seem to get rid of these excess pounds—and I could tell the severe toll they were starting to take on my health.

My doctor tried to help me lose weight with prescribed medications. I tried one prescription after another, but none of them ever worked. I would lose some weight, and then gain it all back, plus more. I also tried many exercise programs, stints of swimming at the YMCA, and exercise programs at the local recreation center, and I even bought a treadmill. The only useful result of this exercise was to make me stronger, and strengthen my cardiovascular system. However, I never lost any "real" weight.

I tried NutriSystem, Slim-Fast, Richard Simmons's Deal-A-Meal, Ayds chocolate hunger suppression "candy," Atkins, the Scarsdale diet, the grapefruit diet, the all-fruit diet, the Caveman diet, and then the new and improved Atkins diet (I never thought I could get sick of too much sausage or meat, but trust me, I did). I was even put under hypnosis, but although it was relaxing, it didn't seem to have any lasting effect. I have tried many, many weight loss strategies to the best of my ability to lose this excess weight. Nothing ever worked—one failure after another.

On my fiftieth birthday, during my yearly physical exam, my new doctor informed me that I was the proud recipient of type 2 adult onset diabetes. I guess the Lord does have a sense of humor! When I added that to my growing list of health challenges—my painful outbreaks of gout; hip, knee, and joint inflammation and pain; and my obstructive sleep apnea—I was starting to despair of *ever* being able to take off my excess weight the normal way. After all, I was exercising, I wasn't eating sugar, and I was watching what I ate. What more could I do? I just never seemed to be able to lose any significant amount of weight. My frustration and desperation grew accordingly.

My doctor firmly insisted that I do three things, immediately: 1) stop eating sugar, or any products that have sugar in any of the first four ingredients listed on the label; 2) cut way back on my carb intake; and 3) find some kind of exercise that I could and would do daily and religiously. I followed his instructions explicitly (much to his surprise) and within three months my blood sugar levels had returned to normal, with an average weekly reading of 117, and my cholesterol levels were within the accepted norms.

My doctor was quite pleased with my commitment and follow-through, and I have been following his regime for three years now. I dusted off my trusty old bicycle once again to deal with my diabetes, now weighing in at 375 pounds. My trusty old Schwinn gave me a renewed sense of self-worth, as well as a sense of mobility, of fleetness not usually associated with someone of my heft. I was strong and could ride for miles. (I originally thought that I would ride around the block, but that has since turned into an 8,000+ miles per year routine for me!) The more I rode, the better I felt; the better I felt, the more I rode. What a cycle (no pun intended)!

However, while I did lose some weight initially, what I lost mainly were inches! I was still at 350 pounds (actually, my weight fluctuated between 340 and 360), but I had stopped eating sugar, watched my carb intake, and I rode a bicycle twenty miles a day, rain or shine.

I felt pretty good about myself, and about what I was doing to improve my health. I was controlling my type 2 diabetes; my obstructive sleep apnea was being dealt with by my use of the CPAP (continuous positive air pressure) device, which forced air down my throat to keep the passage open and keep me breathing; and I considered my daily aches and pains as the normal results of my physical activity. I watched what I ate like a proverbial hawk, I rode my bicycle and lifted my weights daily, and while I physically felt in shape, I knew that I still needed to get rid of the 150–200 pounds of excess fat that had been following me around (and lately, catching up with me).

Then one day, all my numbers seemed to spike, and my doctor sent me to see an endocrinologist. Dr. Nyak had me pegged from the moment I walked into his office. He was certain that my pancreas was failing and that *I needed to lose 200 pounds right away*. He emphasized that I needed to lose my excess weight *immediately*, or else my weight-related afflictions would leave me horizontal with around-the-clock bed care within a couple of years. I was too young to be a full-term bed-care patient!

Dr. Nyak stated his medical opinion that I would benefit greatly from weight loss surgery. He was convinced that most—if not all—of my complications from diabetes would be alleviated with the loss of the excess weight. No more diabetes, no more sleep apnea, no more gout, and no more bone spurs. No more trips to five different doctors for test after test after test. This was a dream that captured my imagination and interest!

He suggested that I consider gastric bypass—a form of weight loss surgery—and set me up to see a bariatric surgeon. I had no second thoughts about this. If I did nothing, I would die a painful early death and yet, if I proceeded with surgery, there was a real possibility that there might be complications. So I decided to carefully explore this possibility. I discussed it with my wife, and she expressed some reservations. But I decided that if I were going to die, it was going to be on *my terms*, tackling the problem head on, and not just lying back and accepting this. Cajuns like me are a bit temperamental about going down without a fight!

At this point in my life, what mattered to me most (besides getting rid of this excess weight) was the chance to resume a somewhat normal life for my family and me. My kids were growing, and would soon be on their own, and I really wanted to be fully alive, active, and present for them—to be a grandfather, and to be a husband for my wonderful wife. I had spent all my adult life trying to lose weight. I was now at the very edge of complete disability and had reached a point where *everything* was an effort.

I work for a wonderful city, and their health insurance covered just about every single dime of my weight loss surgery, except for a $150 co-pay, which I was more than glad to pay! My bariatric surgeon and his office staff were instrumental in guiding me through the approval process. They told me what I needed to do, what letters to get, and when they needed them. I gathered and completed the paperwork and they submitted it.

At times some of the insurance company's requirements seemed senseless, but I followed through, made a checklist for myself, as well as a timeline. I also made duplicate copies of everything. I was totally honest with the insurance company, and told them that I firmly believed, as did my doctors, that without this surgery, they would be paying for my care as a 24/7 bed-care patient for the rest of my life. If they were smart, I suggested, they could pay for the surgery, improve my health, and prolong my life. Before the surgery, I usually made at least one weekly visit to some doctor for some weight-related ailment. I did the footwork; I followed through; and my surgery was approved.

I had an open Roux-en-Y (gastric bypass) on Nov. 10, 2003, and my life changed forever!

Today, ten months after my surgery, my life has made a complete 180-degree change in direction and has been transformed! So far I have lost 163 pounds. I had a 66" waist, and it's now 36". I went from a 6XL shirt to a Large. I am no longer a "working diabetic"; that is, I take no medications, but I still don't eat sugar or many carbs. My gout and the pancreatitis are history. My sleep apnea and my knee, hip, and joint pains have disappeared. My life is now centered on proper nutrition and exercise on a regular daily basis. While I am certainly no athlete, I do keep a pretty strict exercise regimen: 20 miles of bicycling a day; 30 minutes of weight lifting (light weights, numerous repetitions); 3–5 miles of jogging, running, walking, and/or rollerblading; 2 miles of rowing; a mile or more of swimming; and I have just added kayaking to my growing array of exercise options.

Immediately after my surgery, I started walking, as the doctor ordered, first across the room, then down the hallway, and eventually down to the end of the block. Then it was off to the races for me. I was walking a mile a day ten days after surgery, then two miles. I kept setting and achieving small and achievable goals. One thing led to another, and I kept adding to my exercise routines.

Before the surgery, I would wake up, drink a pot of coffee, read the paper, fix some breakfast, and spend an hour or two getting ready for work. Now that I don't really "eat" breakfast, I have part of a protein shake, and then head for the gym or the ocean and spend those hours exercising—not to build up muscle, but to tone what I have and to try to keep the "saggage" at bay. Now I find that I get a little edgy and irritable if I don't have my morning workout. I still don't drink caffeinated coffee or beverages. If I have time, I will have some fruit and yogurt, or something high in protein. This really sets me up for the day, and my exercise regimen has become something I actually look forward to with excitement. How my life has changed since my surgery!

Now, ten months out, the only time I see the doc is for a quick-once over, to make sure that I am following the guidelines and sticking to my plan. In fact, I have yet to take any single pill for anything, other than my daily vitamin supplements (not even a headache). I would call that a wonderful reversal of fortune!

Since my surgery, I can honestly say that head hunger has not been an issue for me. I think that my presurgery, diabetic eating plan took care of that little problem early on. Cut out the sugar, and reduce my simple carbs, and most of my hunger disappears. By maintaining a strict adherence to the "pouch rules," and using the *protein first* guidelines, I have not had to address emotional eating issues.

Do I ever experience cravings? Of course I do. Sometimes I crave something crunchy, so I satisfy that with a few soy crisps, and some hummus, with an added dash of protein powder to it. There are times when I yearn for something sweet—so I fix some sugar-free butterscotch pudding, and add a spoon or two of protein powder to it. I make my salads with fresh alfalfa sprouts and Roma tomatoes, add some crumbled feta cheese, and make a light vinaigrette dressing. I satisfy my cravings, but I make sure that my substitutions always follow the *protein first* rule. So far, it's worked for nearly ten months, and still seems to do the job, meet my needs, and keep me on track.

Yes, it's been difficult for me to achieve my weight loss and maintenance goals. It sure wasn't an easy passage for the first several weeks and months. As soon as I returned home from the hospital, I found that I hated the prescribed pain medications. They gave me freaky nightmares, with story lines that would have kept Stephen King writing for decades!

When I arrived home from the hospital, everything felt numb, or else generally painful. I had to deal with sleeplessness, waking up several times each night from either the nightmares or the pain and discomfort. It seemed so unfair that I had to smell all these odors of food being prepared, but couldn't eat or taste anything. Often, during those sleepless nights, my doubts would creep in and spook me. *Why are you doing this to yourself?* But the Creator was wise when he created the sunrise! I was sleeping in our sunroom after my surgery, at the back of the house, and the veil of the night would lift, ever so slowly, and color would start to seep into the landscape. The birds would sing, the crickets would chirp, and the squirrels would chatter away, and life would begin again, just as it did the morning before!

So I resolved, then and there, that I would always wait until the next day to regret anything, or to reach any judgments or conclusions about this surgery. It is too easy to make poor judgment calls in the dark of night, when I know that a beautiful sunrise will always win out for me.

I couldn't deny my difficulties. Dealing with my new internal plumbing took some getting used to and adjustments—the gurgling, rumbling stomach, the changes in how I processed foods, dealing with the occasional "Technicolor yawn," or the gas or changed patterns of bowel movements. I always tried to step back and look at what was going on inside of me and to ask the right questions. What had changed? Had I eaten something unusual or in an unusual fashion?

What was making me sick, queasy, or ill? Usually I could tell why something didn't feel right, and usually it was because I had ignored the little voice in my head that said, "I wouldn't eat that if I were you."

Initially there seemed to be many things that I considered wrong with the progress of my recovery, but between the good folks on the Internet boards and the doctor's staff, I could usually find an answer or a reason as to why things were or were not working. Knowledge and acceptance proved to be powerful coping tools for me.

One major obstacle for me was the voice in my head telling me, "You need to eat, and it has to be right now!" I responded to myself as my bariatric surgeon suggested: "Don't worry about being hungry, and don't worry about not eating; you are literally carrying around 200 pounds of groceries inside your body. You have protein and liquids stored up, and your body has all the nutrition it needs. This is the time to burn up the fat reserves that you have been storing for your entire life!"

After my fourth month of post-op recovery, my life after WLS became quite easy, so long as I maintained my routines, paid attention to the pouch rules, and watched what I ate. I could not have succeeded as well as I have without the love, care, and support of my beautiful wife. I realized that she was facing some difficult challenges of her own in supporting my post-op recovery. We have three older children, and they were certainly not going to eat what I was eating, and vice versa. My wife also comes from farm stock, and one of her greatest joys in life is cooking a meal and seeing it enjoyed, especially by me. Now, I'm not eating *everything* she cooks, and when I do eat, it is in very tiny portions. I think that has bothered her a bit.

She has also struggled with how self-centered I had to become after my surgery. I literally monitored every calorie and every ounce of food. I am fanatical about logging my caloric intake, and I carefully keep count of protein and carbs consumed, vitamins, and so on. I know I am being self-centered, but I have to be, because life after weight loss surgery requires a whole new way of looking at food and dealing with it.

My wife also grew weary of my rapidly diminishing clothes sizes. Every week, I would make another trip to the thrift store and pick up a couple of pairs of pants and a couple of shirts. I was perfectly willing to alter the items myself, but she wanted to be part of the process, so she insisted that she be the one to hem the pants. However, my wife hates to sew! She soon grew frustrated that as soon as she hemmed my new pairs of pants, I had already reduced to a smaller size! I was perfectly willing to use duct tape, but she wouldn't hear of it.

The only other sticky point came when I began to approach her weight, and then proceeded to lose more until I weighed less than she did. Not much was said about this, but we definitely experienced some degree of unspoken tension about that difficult time. She used to remark that she didn't want me weighing less than she did, and it was all done in jest, but I think that the reality of my losing so much, so fast, and so "effortlessly" bothered her on some levels, when she struggled to lose a few pounds here and there.

My kids have taken all this in very good stride. One of my most intense *aha* moments came when my daughter walked downstairs one spring morning and hugged me, as she usually did. She drew back and said, "Oh my God! I can put my arms around you and touch my fingers!"—something she had never been able to do before now.

I'd be satisfied with any weight that had a "1" in front of it—say 199 or 189! Slowly, but surely, my family members are seeing that "protein first" and small portions are a mainstay of my new lifestyle, and they have actually begun to follow suit on most occasions. Now, whenever I make a fresh glass of vegetable juice, or a protein smoothie, they are willing to give it a taste. They may not want one of their own, but they are willing to give Dad's new concoction a try. That is most definitely progress!

My family and friends—and even co-workers—have been supportive and positive. I've heard plenty of horror stories about support from others being lacking, but I feel very fortunate that I have not had to deal with that aspect during my pre- or post-op experience.

My rules for WLS success are pretty simple and straightforward. I have tried to simplify my plan to a few essential guidelines, which makes it easier for me to comply:

- Get rid of all processed sugars in my daily food (or as much as possible).

- Stop the intake of caffeine, in any form (sodas, coffee, tea), and find good healthy alternatives (including plenty of water).

- Don't eat *anything white!* This will eliminate nearly all the bad carbs that are so abundant in store-bought or restaurant food. I don't consume white bread (I use whole wheat instead), white pastas, flours, crackers, and so on. I will allow cauliflower, apples, pears, and cheeses, but nothing overtly white and not nutritionally packed!

My advice about considering weight loss surgery:

- Research all options, and keep a journal.

- Be prepared for major changes in life, including everything from clothing sizes to shopping to relationships. Preparing for changes leads to fewer surprises.

- Find a good on-line support group (like AMOS at www.obesityhelp.com) and attend your local support meetings as much as possible.

- Delve deeply and fearlessly into personal issues to determine if there are other realistic options, or if weight loss surgery is the best and only chance to lose the excess weight. Serious doubts or reservations may indicate the desire to postpone a decision. A person *must* enter this surgery with both eyes wide open. Any doubts should be addressed, and if needed, professional help should be sought.

- Exercise will *have to* become a daily routine to help both mind and body transform.

My weight loss surgery has been one of the most difficult things I have ever done—not impossible, but most definitely difficult. It was not a quick fix, but it works, and works well, if I'm willing to do the work required to really and substantially change my relationship and habits with food, as well as my whole lifestyle. This is a life-changing and life-altering procedure. Without major lifestyle and behavioral changes, I know that I will return to old habits and sabotage my surgery.

I feel great thrills, benefits, and results from my surgery. They include the loss of most of my excess weight; my ability to actually exercise on a regular and vigorous basis; being able to go into any store and buy something off the rack; knowing that I will be around to enjoy my wife and kids for many years to come; and going to see the doctor once a year because I should, and not because *I have to!*

This surgery and the accompanying healing and relearning process have been the most amazing journey that I have ever undertaken in my life! I have been around the world, ridden from pole to pole on two wheels, played for kings and entertained brigands, 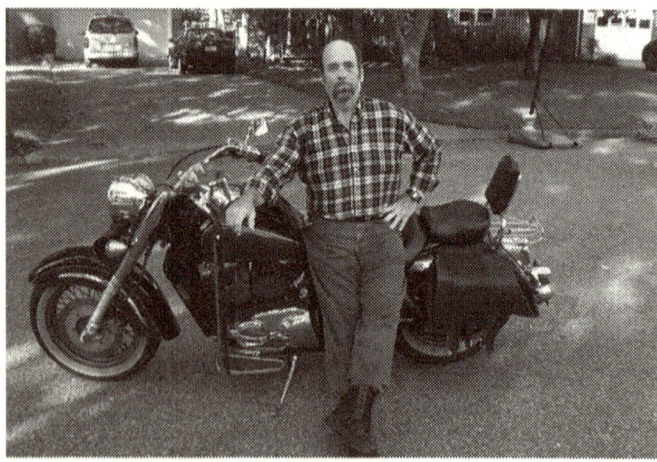 and performed on major stages and small back porches. But *nothing* has come close to the feeling of exhilaration that I get nowadays when I am out and about, almost "normal" in size, eating healthy, and continuing to lose weight! Even if I knew that I had to do this every five years, I would still go through the risk and the pain to maintain this feeling. I am excited to explore this new and amazing second chance at life that WLS has given me.

9

My Yo-Yo Life

by
Marianne McGlaun

I've struggled with my weight for at least fifty of my fifty-four years. I'm only 5'1", and my weight has ranged from an adult low of 112 to a high of 262. I became trapped in a yo-yo dieting pattern of up and down, success and failure, loss and regain. I've tried calorie counting, liquid protein, grapefruit, bananas and milk, low-carb/high-protein, high-carb/ low-protein, Weight Watchers, Overeater's 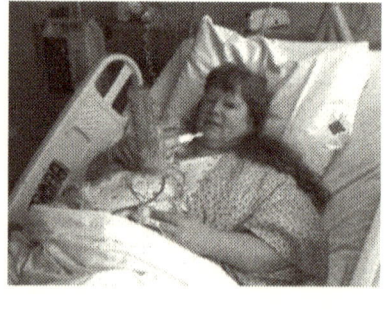 Anonymous, Atkins, counseling, and other weight management programs.

During each successful weight loss, I'd ride the swell of euphoria accompanying lower numbers on the scale, but, during each failure—and my diets always ended in unwelcome failure—I felt the self-criticism that comes with each pound regained.

My lifetime of yo-yo dieting led to health problems that eventually became my comorbidities (life-threatening conditions) associated with all those excess pounds I was never able to lose permanently. For the most part, friends and family accepted me as I was, but it was hard for *me* to accept myself. During my "heavy eras," my weight became a barrier to relationships, activities, and professional growth. My "light eras" were fleeting. They lasted only long enough to make me yearn for them once they vanished almost immediately after their attainment.

I balked at weight loss surgery when it was first recommended, but I was fortunate to have good guidance and support as I made my decision. I'm one of the lucky ones who has had relatively little difficulty with WLS. My decision to have the procedure ranks in the top five best choices I've made in my life. I've now lost all my excess weight and am looking forward to a very long, healthy life to enjoy my new-and-improved body. Here's the story of how I got from *there to here.*

My battle with my excess weight, and eventually my morbid obesity, began as a young child. My dad often took movies of my brother and me growing up in Texas, and the films show that, by age four, I was already getting chubby. My mom put me on my first diet—eggs and tomatoes—when I was seven, so I learned early that dieting was going to be a staple of my life. Despite my mom's best and continued efforts, I stayed overweight through childhood. By my teenage years, however, I began counting calories to keep my weight under control. Surprisingly, during my four years of high school, I stayed between 125 and 135 pounds, and pictures from that time would never suggest that I was a WLS patient-in-waiting.

The next thirty-five years, however, consisted of a roller coaster of events, decisions, and stresses, with the resultant weight gains and losses that accompanied each. As a young adult, I ate my way through a disappointing, but thankfully short, marriage. During those three years, my weight reached a high of 195, even though I was counting calories and taking over-the-counter weight loss pills. I was unhappy and turned to food to fill my lonely personal void and to numb the pain of my troubled marriage.

After I divorced at age twenty-two, I returned to college and focused on my studies, to the complete exclusion of weight management efforts. By my senior year, I tipped the scales at 225. Fortunately, the university I attended required four credits in physical education, so one quarter I signed up for racquetball. I actually enjoyed the sport and continued with it almost daily until graduation. The excess weight put a heavy burden on my knees, but somehow I managed to avoid any long-lasting consequences. My college years were blessed with good friends who apparently overlooked my enormous size.

Upon graduation from college in 1975, I moved to Wyoming to take my first full-time job. I was fortunate to develop some very good friendships and an honest-to-goodness social life. My weight began to drop from 225 to the mid-100s. I'm sure my social life and weight loss fed off each other (pardon the pun). I enjoyed dancing, hiking, and dating. I managed my weight mostly through counting calories and staying active. I was generally pleased with my weight and how I felt about myself.

In 1980, at a weight of 168, I married my second husband. Even though this marriage was more agreeable than the first, my weight rose to 246 pounds during our first three years together, and my weight gain became a major issue in our marriage. At that point, my husband was diagnosed with dangerously high cholesterol levels, so I learned to cook healthier, low-fat foods and gladly adopted them for my own eating program (although, unfortunately, my husband did not). The changes in my meal plan brought my weight down to 190. But that wasn't enough to keep the marriage going. In 1985 I once again divorced.

This time, though, I took the bull by the horns. I was actually anorexic for about two months after the split, eating only half a slice of toast for breakfast, an apple for lunch, and a salad for dinner. I certainly don't condone my strategy, but it did kick my weight loss into hyperdrive. I dropped from 190 to 125 in seven months and stayed there until my move to Washington state the following summer.

In Washington, I lived with a good friend and started a new job. Under the stresses of new surroundings (note the pattern here), my weight once again began to climb, reaching 215 in 1988. My weight control efforts included counseling, counting calories, joining Overeaters Anonymous, and beginning a minimal walking program. My weight varied between the mid- to the upper-100s again for the next five years.

In 1993, I moved to a different town to reenter the teaching field. This was the most miserable year of my professional life! But this time, rather than gaining weight (as usual) in response to the stress, I began *losing* weight. Looking back, my weight loss seemed slow, methodical, and healthy, but I later realized that it was anything but healthful! I only taught one year before switching to a college administration position. In both roles I was a workaholic, averaging 60–80 hours per week. Nevertheless, I managed to continue my minimal walking program and to maintain my slow weight loss. The stress I experienced felt like the good kind of stress, and I truly loved my work.

In March 1997, "the World According to Marianne" came to an abrupt end. I was diagnosed with type 2 diabetes, which explained the weight loss and a number of other changes that had been happening over the previous four years. My doctor had me try several different oral diabetes medications, but none worked for more than a few weeks or months. In 1998 my doctor finally convinced me to begin taking insulin injections. It felt like a death sentence to me—the death of my freedom to do/live/be/eat as I wished.

An unanticipated result of my insulin use was an immediate and dramatic reversal in my weight loss. I gained thirty pounds per year, going from 112 pounds in 1998 to 262 pounds in 2003—a steady and unstoppable gain of 150 pounds in five years. I was mad at my body for crippling me with this wretched disease—and at myself for not realizing sooner what was happening.

During the five years after I started injecting insulin, I had changed doctors a few times and had pleaded with each for a prescription of a weight-loss medication to counteract the weight gain caused by my insulin use. The doctor I began seeing in 2001 asked me if I had ever considered weight loss surgery instead of a "diet pill." I felt *insulted*. How dare he think that I'd need such a drastic remedy for a problem that could easily be resolved with a simple diet pill!

Every three months when I saw him for diabetes follow-up, he would suggest the procedure again. Frankly, I was getting angry with his nagging. But nag he did, for a full eighteen months, until I finally decided to research the procedure. I was sure I'd find enough bad press on WLS to convince my doctor that it was *not* the right option for me. I also just knew I could lose the weight on my own. (Of course, my inner certainty had never yet changed the arc of my yo-yo.)

As I started researching the surgery, I was surprised to learn that many type 2 diabetics have achieved freedom from insulin and/or oral medications *within days or months* of their bariatric surgery. I needed more confirmation, so I contacted over 100 bariatric surgeons to ask what kind of results their patients with type 2 diabetes had experienced. I received replies from doctors at some of the most prestigious medical facilities in the country, including Duke University Hospital and Mt. Sinai Medical Center. Every surgeon who responded confirmed what I had learned in my research. I began to believe that WLS might actually be the right decision for me. I began to get excited about the possibilities.

I was also surprised and thrilled to learn that WLS has a phenomenal track record of improving other dangerous medical conditions, including high blood pressure. In 2002 my doctor had started me on blood pressure medication because my in-office readings were consistently above normal. While oral medication for high blood pressure was less of an intrusion upon my life than insulin injections for diabetes, I began to understand that WLS could give me the biggest bang for my buck. I also began to understand the full array of benefits I could derive from looking better, feeling more confident, and ending my vicious cycle of yo-yo dieting that had plagued me since high school.

By chance, I found a local WLS support group in May 2003. At the first meeting I attended, I met a woman who was scheduled for Roux-en-Y gastric bypass surgery three weeks later. Since my eyesight is so impaired from my diabetes that I do not drive out of town, I asked if I could ride with her to her pre-op appointment the following month. She graciously agreed, and I was fortunate to get an appointment on the same date in June 2003. The staff at the WISH Center answered the many questions I could not get answered in my research, and the surgeon thoroughly explained his approach to the procedure. I knew I had come to the right place.

I made my decision in June 2003 to have WLS. Although my insurance would not cover any cosmetic procedure, I decided to pursue an exception since the procedure would also effectively treat my diabetes. My doctor provided a powerful written recommendation for the surgery, which the insurance company immediately denied. I then began the appeal process, submitting a ream of documentation (including medical journal articles, the responses from the bariatric surgeons I had contacted, analysis of costs for WLS compared to the costs of treating diabetic complications, testimonials of type 2 diabetes patients whose condition resolved with WLS, etc.).

Each time I sent an appeal package, it was denied within one to three days. I wondered if the bean counters at the insurance company were even bothering to read the material I was sending.

The final step in the appeal process was a face-to-face meeting with representatives of the insurance company. I was permitted to bring my own team: an attorney specializing in medical cases, a registered nurse/college nursing educator, and a personal friend of twenty-five years who well knew my health history. This meeting was scheduled, of all days, on the exact day I had initially scheduled my surgery in August. I saw that coincidence as an omen. Each person on my team thought our presentation was well received and that, just maybe, we had penetrated the bureaucratic barriers and touched the collective reasonability of the insurance representative. One week later I received their final denial, dated on the same day as our meeting. Apparently, we had made no dent whatsoever in the brick-wall mentality of corporate medical insurance.

I immediately called the WISH Center to select another surgery date in late October. As a new facility, the center had offered reduced rates during its first six months in operation. They were able to squeeze me in so that I could take advantage of this window of opportunity. The hospital where the surgery would take place also extended their reduced rate until my rescheduled surgery date, and permitted me to arrange payments over a twelve-month period, interest free. I could handle the financial arrangements, and I justified the expense in this way: the cost would be no more than for a good, new car, and I was willing to pay that price for a "vehicle" I could "drive" for the rest of my life!

Between June and October, I religiously followed the WISH Center's pre-op practice program. I was required to journal everything I ate, my daily exercise, the supplements I took, the liquids I drank, and my awareness of what I was doing. Journaling is an activity I despise, so it took a lot of commitment to follow through as thoroughly as I did. Although I did not understand it at first, the goal of the activity was not to achieve weight loss, but rather to achieve awareness of the changes that inevitably accompany the surgery.

The emphasis was on protein, supplements, and water consumption, along with vigorous exercise. At first I tried to eat tiny portions and felt starved all day and night. So I called the WISH Center, and my nutritionist explained that I could eat as much as I wanted as long as I followed their nutrient guidelines. During this precious time, I reeducated myself, changed my eating habits, and even lost twenty-two pounds in the process! Once my commitment was established, I never felt deprived, restless, unsure, or indecisive. I knew I was on the right track and that I had made the perfect decision for me.

It was only four days before the surgery that I allowed myself to feel the depth and intensity of my excitement over my imminent emancipation. I honestly never felt fear or trepidation. I was more afraid of *not* having the surgery than of having it, because of my deteriorating health conditions.

Early on the morning of October 21, I arrived at the hospital feeling neither dread nor excitement—just confidence. The most difficult part of the initial procedure, as with all the other surgeries I've had, was the IV, because my hands have tiny, rolling veins. But once the intravenous tube was in, I was ready to get on with it. I sang a little song over and over in my head and shared it with my surgical team (to the tune of "Oh, What a Beautiful Morning"):

> *"With a 10/21-derful surgeon,*
> *On this 10/21-derful day,*
> *This 10/21-derful patient*
> *Has everything going her way!"*

The last thing I remember was smiling at one of the surgical nurses. Then I awoke in the recovery room. It was not, however, a pleasant awakening. It was dry heaves that revived me—probably not the best physical activity for a gastric bypass patient with a brand new five-inch hole in her belly. Passing in and out of awareness, I somehow ended up in my private room on the new bariatric surgery ward.

I felt miserable, the IV hurt, the nausea didn't subside, and my kidneys were barely functioning. Over my three-day stay in the hospital, I gained close to thirty pounds of water weight, pushing my weight to an estimated 270 pounds.

The surgeon finally put me on a diuretic on the third day, and that evening the dam broke. I filled that little bag over and over again, but only eliminated about five pounds of the water gain. Upon release from the hospital on day four, I could hardly sit up in the wheelchair. I felt and looked like the Pillsbury Doughboy!

For the next ten days after I got out of the hospital, I stayed with my best friend/support person, who is surely the world's best nurse. He took care of my every need, including the suppositories I needed for the nausea. It took eight days after surgery for the nausea to disappear, and those eight days were almost unbearable at times. I actually felt worse once I got to my friend's house than I had felt in the hospital. I remember huddling under a blanket as I painfully walked around the house as recommended to prevent blood clots, feeling that I was literally dragging the weight of the world with me. I moaned with every step and could hardly wait to sit down again, only to find that I was just as miserable sitting. During those eight days, the food ads on TV made me gag, and I really struggled to get down my liquid diet. It felt like my misery would never end.

Finally, late on the eighth day, the nausea subsided and I began to feel better. I even began to enjoy the liquid diet I was required to maintain for the first two weeks. Within another couple of days, I found that I craved anything protein. I faithfully drank my protein drinks, vegetable broth, and water in the small sips recommended. I even bought a bottle of clear clam juice because it had just a hint of protein. It was amazing to me that it could actually take me 30 minutes to sip four ounces of liquid!

During those first two weeks post-op, amazing changes began to take place. By my two-week appointment, I had lost all the water weight gain, an incredible drop from my peak weight of 270 in the hospital. As if that weren't enough, I was off blood pressure medication by the end of the first week, and had lowered my insulin requirement by 70%!

When my best friend returned me to my home eighteen days after my surgery, I weighed 227. I was already into the four-week pureed foods phase of my meal plan and enjoyed baby food even more than I had as an infant. Alright, it got a little boring by the fourth week of this phase, but it still wasn't as bad as I had expected. I made a point of selecting a wide variety of foods and found that I could eat almost anything pureed, including many meats. My friends complained that the fish and vegetable puree combination smelled like cat food!

I insisted on eating fish daily, not just for its protein, but because I had read about its preventative effect on hair loss. During my entire recovery process, I never lost any hair, which was great, since I'm very vain about my hair. Today, one year after surgery, I still eat a quarter-cup of cold-water fish at least six days a week. My choices range from canned tuna and mackerel to fresh salmon and halibut.

It didn't take long for my co-workers to start noticing a difference in my appearance. I had told only a select few before the surgery because I didn't want to hear any negative comments. By the end of 2003, I had lost sixty-eight pounds. Some folks even asked if I was ill. I was delighted to tell them that I was the healthiest I had been in years, and to then share my secret. To my surprise and delight, no one rained on my parade. Seeing the amazing results for themselves defused any skepticism.

Sometimes I tend to put on blinders when I have a clear goal and a clear path to achieve it. Such was the case with my weight loss after my WLS. I committed myself totally to reaching my goal within that 12- to 18-month window of opportunity, when the chance of losing 100% of excess weight is at its greatest. *Nothing* deterred my drive. I was able to focus completely on my goal, and my pace was as furious as my determination was fierce.

Of course, I enjoyed a luxury that most WLS patients don't have: I have no obligations outside myself: no husband, boyfriend, children or grandchildren, pets, housemate, and no one to influence my eating choices or exercise routines. I reached my goal, not in 12–18 months, but in 9 months and 9 days after surgery! On July 30, 2004, my talking scale said the words I'd been waiting a lifetime to hear: "Your weight is 123 pounds."

Yes, 123 pounds. That may sound like an odd goal, but January 23 is my birthday, and I've always wanted to weigh my birthday. I've reached that weight precious few times in my adult life, but have never stayed there for long. This time, though, it is both real *and* permanent!

For another month, I pursued an additional five-pound loss, just so that I could have some wiggle room as I began to stabilize my weight. I ended up losing another eight pounds, down to 115, by late August. At that point, I knew I had to stop losing, and start learning how to maintain a very comfortable weight that would never again exceed 123 pounds.

During the entire time that I was losing weight, I followed the same guidelines that any other dieter (WLS patient or not) has to follow to succeed. I ate what was on my meal plan, gradually increased my exercise program, drank my water and other liquids, and sought the support of friends. The only difference is that this time I had the WLS *tool* to help me.

I have had four simple rules for WLS success:

1.   Commitment

2.   Commitment

3.   Commitment

4.   Commitment

I've made, and kept, my commitments to 1) my meal plan, 2) my supplement and liquid consumption, 3) my exercise program, and 4) my targets and goals. For me, it's been critically important to *put myself first* for however long it takes to reach my weight loss and maintenance goals. I constantly strive to remember: just because I have "the tool" doesn't mean that I can take this job lightly. These are my guidelines.

• *Slow down!* I'm amazed at how fast I used to eat. These days, I watch those around me vacuum down their food as if it's going to escape if they don't consume it at lightning speed. I now take at least twenty, and preferably thirty or more, minutes to eat each of my small meals and snacks. It takes twenty minutes or more for my stomach to begin to feel full.

• *Take tiny bites.* The larger my bite, the more quickly I eat. I cut a three-inch link sausage into at least fifteen pieces, then take two bites for each piece. I can easily take 20–25 bites from a single soda cracker or eat a single green bean at a time.

• *Chew, chew, chew!* This also helps lengthen the time it takes me to eat a meal or snack, and also better prepares the food for my stomach pouch.

• *When eating out, I request side orders or ask for special orders.* I have no problem explaining my situation to food servers in restaurants and find that most of them are both fascinated and eager to help.

• *I use chewable or liquid supplements every day to ensure that my body has adequate and balanced nutrition.*

• *I keep myself well hydrated.* I force myself to consume two cups of filtered water each day. Then the rest of my liquid consumption consists of decaffeinated coffee, herbal tea, sugar-free uncarbonated beverages, and sugar-free Popsicles or gelatin (yep, they count as liquids). Sometimes I forget to drink my liquids, but usually I'm working on a cup of something wet between each meal or snack. I have found that liquid is probably the most important nutrient when it comes to promoting consistent weight loss.

- *I exercise daily.* Even at my heaviest, I would drag myself onto my treadmill each morning for an incredibly slow thirty-minute walk of less than one mile and feel exhausted afterward. But walk I did. I felt even lousier when I didn't walk than when I did. My walk today is still thirty minutes in length, but I'm at double the pace (3.5 mph). I bought a treadmill so that I can walk indoors, rain or shine, and I actually miss my treadmill when I'm sick or away from home. I'm *not* a morning person, so I climb on my treadmill right after I rise in the morning, before I become conscious enough to realize what I'm doing. By the time I finish a thirty-minute walk and hit the shower, I'm just about ready to wake up and face the day, *and* I've completed my aerobic commitment to myself! A friend convinced me to add some form of weight training to my exercise program. Three months after surgery, I purchased a set of resistance bands and began with the lightest band for a two-circuit, twenty-minute workout, which I do six days a week. I'm toying with the idea of joining a gym, not just for the physical benefits but also for the social interactions.

- I *never ever* lose sight of my goal, or stop working to achieve it.

From time to time, now that I've reached my goal weight, I experiment with a little extra food volume. Most of the time, I can easily get away with a couple extra tablespoons at a meal or snack, but sometimes even that small addition will come right back up, especially if I eat too fast. In an effort to minimize eating too rapidly, I try to take a minimum of twenty minutes to eat a meal or snack.

The good news is that I apparently haven't stretched my stomach pouch during the year since my surgery. The bad news is that I never know when or if the extra bit of food will stay down or not. But these challenges are minor inconveniences that give me no appreciable concern, even if they continue for the rest of my life.

I realized at the very end of my race (as I neared my goal) that the stomach cramps I experienced from time to time weren't caused by the food I was eating; instead, they were caused by the food I was *not* eating. I wasn't eating enough and my stomach pouch would go into spasms because it wanted more food. Listening to my body is not something I'm used to doing, and it will take consistent and prolonged effort to learn to interpret the signals my body is giving me. Now that I've added a little more food in my maintenance phase, the stomach cramps are almost nonexistent.

Although I have no fear that I will ever again regain my excess weight, I now find my biggest challenge is to learn how to *be* a thin person. It's simply true that "fatties" are treated very differently than their thin counterparts. Sales representatives, service personnel, educators, potential dates or partners, and sometimes even friends and family react to me so differently (and positively) as a thin person. I find myself alternating between outrage and delight, between resentment and celebration. I still struggle to become accustomed to hearing myself described as "skinny, svelte, tiny, thin, and slim."

And I still struggle with relationships. My relationship with food had always been that of "best friend"—the friend that was there for me, no matter what. Throughout my life, I allowed only four emotions to drive my overeating: when I was bad, sad, glad, or mad (which I guess just about covers it all). As I yo-yoed between the low-100s and mid-200s, I consoled all the stresses of life—two marriages, two divorces, college, families, jobs, and social events—with food. I allowed my relationship with food and my resulting obesity to keep me from participating in activities that I would have enjoyed.

Relationships with people, on the other hand, have been less comforting. Two failed marriages, along with another failed long-term relationship, dealt a pretty heavy blow to my self-confidence in the relationship arena. The declining self-confidence that accompanied my obesity, together with my low self-esteem, didn't make me a very attractive potential partner. My weight has always been a factor in relationships. Either I was too fat to attract the type of man I dreamed of, or, in the rare times when I was thin, I'd get scared off when a relationship began to develop. I'd put weight back on in order to drive away any man who expressed an interest in me. It's been a vicious circle.

This time, though, I'm thin to stay. I don't and won't have my well-used crutch to lean on when a relationship seems imminent. That is forcing me to explore why I have been unsuccessful at relationships for most of my adult life. I'm sure there are elements of fear involved: fear of intimacy, fear of commitment, fear of rejection, and fear of loss of self. I know I've got a lot of work to do on understanding the connection between weight and relationships, and more beyond that.

In the privacy and solace of my home, I dream of engaging in a fulfilling social life. I want to date and feel confident enough now to risk putting myself "on the market." But it's been so long since I've played the dating game that I've mostly forgotten how to deal the first hand. I've told my work associates and friends that I'm open to dating and willing for them to introduce me to single gentlemen they know. So far, though, no one has offered any introductions. That makes me realize that I must do the work myself, just as I did in deciding to have my WLS and making the commitment to reach my goal in record time. I look forward to the day that I'll meet Mr. Right-for-Me. Today, I know that there's at least a chance.

I know I could fall back into some old habits that would put the pounds back on, but this time there's something different—for one thing, the WLS *tool*—and, for another, the awareness and commitment I've made to this process. I really haven't ever experienced anything quite like this before, so the feeling of this success is far more concrete and permanent than at any other point in my life.

From a physical aspect, the improvements have been impressive. When I decided to have the surgery as a way to treat my diabetes, I used 86–120 units of daily insulin, taken in two to five injections a day, and I needed to monitor my blood sugar five or more times each day. In May 2004, seven months after my surgery, my insulin requirements had decreased to the point that I was able to switch to a 24-hour insulin (Lantus). With my egg-sized stomach pouch, I eat so little that the Lantus insulin lasts me all day! I started the Lantus at 17 units, one time a day, but am now down to 8 or 9 units. That's an incredible drop of over 90% in insulin need! My hemoglobin A1C (three-month blood sugar average) was recently a relatively healthy 6.1. I now check my blood sugar only once a day, rather than five or more times, and my readings are almost always normal. These are truly miraculous outcomes for me! And I still have hopes they will improve even more.

The feeling of freedom I have already achieved is phenomenal. I check my blood sugar and inject my insulin first thing every morning. Then, as long as I follow my meal plan—which is *no* inconvenience whatsoever, even when traveling—and get some exercise during the day, I'm *free* until the next morning. These improvements are liberating to my soul and inspiring to my heart.

Reaching my goal-minus-eight weight, I now wear a size 4–6 in both shirts and slacks (it used to be 26–28 or 4X). I easily fit into a 36C bra (formerly 44D) and a size 6 panty (down from 14). Even my shoe size has shrunk from a 6-wide to a 5-regular. My waist measures 27 inches (down from 61) and my hips are 36 inches. It's hard for me to actually believe these tiny numbers are my own measurements.

Daily activities—ranging from personal hygiene to driving to fitting into seats and spaces—are no longer the torturous challenges they used to be. I can bend into any position I need, fasten any kind of belt around me, walk in a model-straight line, cross my legs, dance, prance, and otherwise reach/bend/stoop whenever and however I need or want to. I can now keep going all day long without tiring and am constantly amazed at how much easier it is to do almost everything.

What have been the greatest thrills and benefits of my WLS success?

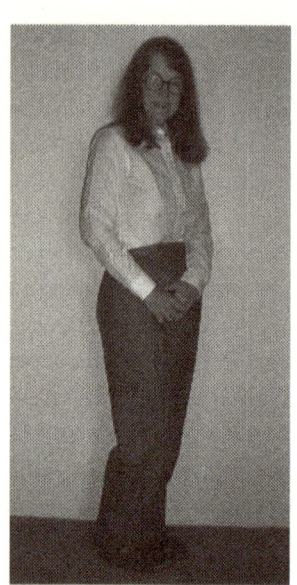

- *Controlling diabetes with minimal intrusion on my life.* The sense of freedom from less need for insulin and monitoring can only be appreciated by those who live with the disease.

- *Shopping in a regular store.* This is both a blessing and a curse. The positive is that clothes fit (in my case, *small* clothes), and the negative is that I buy too many of them (but I save lots of money on food!).

- *Knowing that I'll never have to do this again.* It was expensive, but I bought this incredible WLS *tool* that will help me permanently manage my weight.

- *Looking forward to all the possibilities, especially dating/marriage and a longer/healthier/more productive life to enjoy with someone special.*

- *Getting to know the woman who looks back at me from the other side of the mirror.* Although I'm still surprised when I find her looking at me, she's becoming one of my best friends and it's a real pleasure to get to know her!

I made the right choice when I decided to have weight loss surgery. My risk of dying from the procedure was far less than my risk of dying prematurely from continued obesity or comorbidities (diabetes, high blood pressure, high cholesterol, sleep apnea, etc.). I have never once felt ashamed, intimidated, or inferior that I chose to have WLS to treat diabetes, eliminate high blood pressure, control my weight, bolster my self-image, and transform my body image. My quality of life has been greatly and immediately enhanced. I am proud to tell others why I chose to have weight loss surgery. I couldn't be happier living a yo-yo-free life.

10

My Journey from Fat Guy to Iron Man!

by
Scotty Morrison

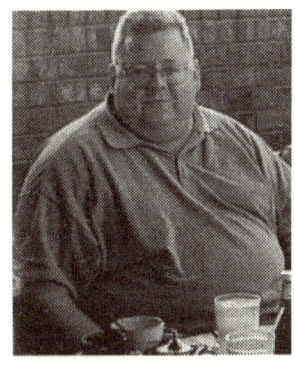

I haven't always struggled with obesity. I was never skinny, but I never stood out as overweight as a child or a teen. But my family warned me that I might experience a major weight gain as a young adult, since this seems to be part of my genetic heritage on both sides of my family. Throughout high school and part of college I was only mildly overweight. However, my family's warnings were prophetic. By the end of college I weighed 220 pounds.

Food has always been a drug that I can abuse. It was always there for me when I felt stressed. I tended to eat until I felt *sedated,* rather than *satiated.* It didn't help that I grew up in a home that experienced its own forms of abuse. My dad abused food and people. My mom abused food, alcohol, and chemicals. Looking back on my childhood, some of the more peaceful, and less insane, moments of my life growing up were when we were preparing food for meals or parties. When things went crazy in our home, I tended to just eat something and stay out of the way. All the warning signs of a looming food addiction were there. I just didn't see them.

My obesity has definitely been an obstacle in my relationships. In my profession as a technologist and engineer, I believe some people discounted my ideas and inputs, simply because of my weight. I think that they may have seen me as lazy and undisciplined in my physical existence, and that their judgments may have spilled over into judgments about my career and/or intellect.

I was quite embarrassed by my size and weight, and this factored into many decisions I made regarding relationships. For example, I chose to miss my ten-year high school reunion because of the reaction I feared from high school friends. I also recall a time at the Phoenix Zoo, when I saw a very close high school buddy about twenty-five yards away. We had been inseparable friends during high school. But I chose, on that day, to avoid speaking to him because I was so ashamed of my weight gain and appearance.

Throughout my twenties and early thirties, my weight problems continued to worsen. A work-related back injury impaired my ability to exercise, and then my particular combination of genetics, bad food choices, and immobility created a vicious circle of weight gain. By my thirty-fifth birthday I weighed more than 315 pounds. As my weight increased, my health took a deep dive downhill. I experienced severe chronic joint and back pain. I also developed obstructive sleep apnea as a complication of my morbid obesity. I became depressed and often suffered from migraines. I prayed for a way to return to health. Nothing seemed to work.

Exercise was not really an option for me in the year or so before my bariatric surgery. My back hurt so bad that almost *any* motion was painful. In early years, I had really enjoyed exercise. In fact, when I first met my wife, Sue, in 1986, I weighed about what I do now. Our earliest dates were bike rides and trips to the gym. However, I injured my back in the late 80s while loading cargo for an airline. Once I hurt my back, my exercise stopped, my food intake stayed constant, and my weight started to surge in a vicious, negative cycle.

I never went on any of the crazy fad diets. But I did try a number of mainstream programs. I tried the Pritikin diet, the Zone diet, the Atkins diet, and also an Opti-fast program under the care of a bariatric physician. Each time I tried a diet, I would lose somewhere between 25–50 pounds, and then regain it all, and usually some more, once I stopped that particular diet plan. In hindsight, I made exactly the wrong choices when I dieted. I would starve myself for two or three days, and then, when my hunger finally drove me back to food, I overconsumed for a few more days until my extreme hunger receded.

After exhausting many attempts to lose my excess weight—including over-the-counter and medically supervised weight management programs—my wife and I made the decision to pursue weight loss surgery with one of Colorado's most experienced bariatric surgeons. In May of 2002, a friend showed me a clipping from our local newspaper. The ad announced that the Greeley Medical Clinic was presenting a seminar on medical alternatives for weight loss. At the time, I weighed 324 pounds, had severe back pain, and was basically miserable with my life. I did attend that seminar, and I believe it changed my life for the better.

During the seminar, Dr. Johnell, the bariatric surgeon, described a number of approaches to weight loss. He spoke about diet/exercise plans, supervised medical programs, and several surgical procedures. The procedure that caught my attention was the Roux-en-Y, or gastric bypass. He clearly identified its potential risks and benefits. *That was the moment that I realized I might actually have some realistic hope for losing my excess weight.*

I was troubled by the fact that a significant proportion of Roux-en-Y gastric bypass patients suffered some sort of negative side effect. I was disturbed to learn that as many as 1 out of every 50 patients die from weight loss surgery (a 2% mortality rate). I was worried that I could potentially be disabled for life, or die from the procedure. Then I did my own reality check and took a searching and fearless look at my life as it was right then. I was already disabled by back pain, headaches, and fatigue. The five-year mortality rate for superobese people like me who did not have WLS was actually higher than for those who did have the surgery! As an engineer, it came down to the numbers. As an emotional being, it came down to a desperate desire to live again.

Over the next several months, I jumped through hoops to qualify for the surgery. I appreciated my conversations with Dr. Johnell, and his insistence that patients be fully informed about the surgery, its risks and benefits, and the lifestyle changes required after undergoing the procedure. He made it clear that the surgery involved very real risks, and that it was *not* a simple, quick, or easy fix for my morbid obesity. His only claim was that WLS might finally give me a very effective and powerful tool to use in my fight. He was right.

I started to get a grasp on my emotional eating issues as I began to prepare for my WLS. My doctor was very clear that the required changes in lifestyle were going to be difficult. The clinic gave its patients a lot of materials and insights to help us prepare for the changes ahead.

My back pain was so bad at this time that I was having epidural spinal injections every 3–4 weeks, along with taking OxyContin. I felt desperate for relief and began to explore the process of scheduling surgery to relieve my back pain. My medical pain specialist suggested that I consider having the gastric bypass as a "prelude" or even alternative to the back surgery. His advice was sound. I never did need that back surgery. Weight loss surgery offered the key to my pain relief.

In preparing for gastric bypass surgery, my doctor provided thorough information about how and what I would eat after the surgery, how I could develop a realistic exercise plan, and how I might handle some of the emotional stresses I could be expected to face. My wife, Sue, and I talked endlessly to satisfy ourselves that the potential benefits of the surgery were well worth the risks. We had four kids, and didn't want to make any quick or uninformed decisions that might cost me my life and my family.

I was fortunate enough to work for a large company that offered choices for medical care, so I was able to find the coverage that would underwrite my weight loss surgery and then moved to that plan during the open enrollment period. I was relentless, refused to take no for an answer, and talked to enough of their staff to find the right openings in their bureaucracy. My procedure was approved.

On August 6, 2003, I had my Roux-en-Y gastric bypass surgery. At 5' 6.5", with a waist size of 60, I had reached an all-time high weight of 332 a couple days after my surgery. However, I had lost eleven pounds by the time I climbed onto the gurney and proceeded with the bariatric surgery that may well have saved my life. My goal that day was to weigh 165 pounds, which was what I weighed as a junior in high school.

Any major surgery has its risks, and weight loss surgery is most definitely major surgery. Unfortunately, I became one of the complications statistics: the day after my gastric bypass, I developed severe abdominal pain. The doctor responded quickly and decisively. He took me back into surgery to fix a leak in my intestines. I woke up in pretty bad shape. I was on a respirator and in considerable pain. During the second surgery, my vital signs got pretty unstable. So I was intubated and had my hands restrained so I would not pull the tube out of my airway when I woke up. This was a really scary time for me, even though the nurses did a good job of explaining what was going on. I felt panic, on top of the pain. I would not wish conscious airway intubation on anybody, *ever*. Thankfully, I was back out of intensive care within a few days. Although it was no fun having two surgeries in two days, I deeply appreciated the skillful care I received throughout my hospital stay.

My ordeal wasn't yet done. I had to keep a rather large drain catheter in place for about a month after the surgery. It was really weird looking down at that thing sticking out from under my sternum—very unpleasant, and quite unnatural. I went through a few days of panic, thinking that I might starve to death. I knew this was irrational, but the emotion was real, and very painful, nonetheless.

My first "workout" was ten days after surgery. I walked down my driveway, and made it to the house next door, but I barely made it back to my house! I just didn't feel very good for about five weeks after the surgery. It was great to be losing weight, but I felt lousy and not at all myself. For financial reasons, I had to go back to work about 2.5 weeks after my surgery. I would have probably done better if I could have rested for another week or so.

About six weeks postsurgery, however, I actually felt pretty good. By that time, I had lost about 50 pounds! My severe back/joint pain and sleep apnea had literally disappeared, and I started going to the gym to begin swimming and moderate weight training. Within four months after surgery, I had virtually no health problems and required no medication!

What was most astounding was how quickly my health returned. I literally felt physically great about ten weeks after my weight loss surgery. My return to a sense of healthiness or well-being was not a process. It was more as if I woke up about two months after WLS and was flat-out surprised at how good I felt. Even though I still had over 100 pounds to lose, that first 60 pounds was what did it for me. It really felt like a turnkey process for me: have the surgery and, so soon, enjoy my new body and feel great!

My doctor insisted that I attend a support group, and it really helped me get through the difficult lifestyle adjustments of following the eating program, doing the exercise, taking the vitamins, and consuming the ever-present protein powder! This really helped me take advantage of the weight loss window of opportunity, or honeymoon. Ten months out from my surgery, I'd lost almost 160 pounds.

I was one of those very fortunate patients who experienced profound satiety for almost a full year after the surgery. This was a great gift, as it gave me kind of a timeout from my previous emotional eating issues. In addition, if I ate too much, I became very uncomfortable physically. So the surgery provided me with both a positive and a negative physical reinforcement mechanism. This really helped me be able to look at my emotional eating issues more objectively, and provided a season wherein I could (and did) learn to enjoy food, rather than abuse it as a drug. The one thing I have had to do is make sure that I don't transfer my addictive tendencies from food to other ingestibles. I found that alcohol became more tempting, and even that old bad habit of chewing tobacco tempted and tested me for a few months.

Most friends were very supportive. Some thought I was taking the "easier way" out, but they also respected that I had carefully thought through the issues, and even consulted many of my friends before making the decision. I did notice that some co-workers were a little jealous about some of my successes. While I didn't self-promote, some people engaged in back-biting when some of my story came out in a front-page article in our local paper. It was really weird to be accused of being "full of myself" or of "thinking I was better than others." It didn't really hurt me; rather, I was just mystified and disillusioned by some people's immature reactions to my successes.

One exciting aspect of my extreme weight loss is that I have been able to return to a former passion—the triathlon. On June 22, 2003, I competed in the Greeley Sprint Triathlon. It was not the Ironman, but doing something like this would have been absolutely impossible for me less than one year earlier!

My recovery has been so complete that this summer I did a three-day bike ride called the Courage Classic, which raises funds for a children's hospital in Denver. The 160-mile ride goes over many of the highest passes in Colorado. It is impossible to express how much my life and health have improved.

I remember suffering a bit as I worked my way up the four-mile climb to the summit—but still having this incredible sense of gratitude that *I had my life back!* And now I realize that the pain of climbing that mountain was actually less than the pain my body (back, joints, headaches, etc.) used to feel when I was super-obese. As I reached the top of the climb, I can literally remember feeling this powerful sense that God told me, "Welcome back!"

I've come to understand that physical exercise is absolutely vital to my well-being—especially in the area of weight training. If I maintain a consistent schedule of moderate full-body weight training, then I have no pain anywhere in my body, I sleep better, and find it very easy to maintain my weight. I'm kind of a "streak" exerciser. If I keep going, it stays easy. If I back off for even a week or so, I can "fall off the wagon" and then must take intentional steps to get restarted. I am training now for the Florida Ironman Triathlon (2.4-mile swim, 112-mile bike, 26.2-mile run) in November 2006. I don't think I can win the thing; I just want to try to push the envelope on my physical performance before my age catches up with me.

I have done a pretty good job of maintaining my vitamin and protein intake. In addition, as my stomach has stretched, I have learned to use a technique called *water loading* to maintain some of the feelings of the little pouch. Water loading is basically drinking 5–6 ounces of cold water approximately twenty minutes before eating. This causes the pouch to gently stretch and sends a satiety signal to the brain. It also causes the pouch openings to slightly contract and give more tone to the pouch—thus accentuating the feeling of fullness when I eat. I try not to let myself get too hungry. If hungry, I will start with a small protein portion, eat that, and then wait 20–30 minutes. If still hungry, I will eat some more, and so on. This enables me to eat whenever I want to, but maintains the smaller pouch.

It is a wonderful thing to have my life back. I am a better husband, father, and friend to those around me. I give thanks to God, my family, and my whole medical team. Their love, skill, caring, and time have, literally, saved and transformed my life.

Losing so much weight has had a huge impact on my relationship with just about everybody in my life. With casual acquaintances, I seem to have disappeared. What I mean is that, when one is very obese, people tend to look and gawk due to curiosity and disgust. I remember having people watch what I bought at the grocery store, or inspect what I was eating while in a restaurant. Sometimes little kids would come up to me and say, "You are fat!" Obviously, most parents would be embarrassed by their children's actions, but usually the little kids just thought I was interestingly different. I was never offended by the honest appraisal of a four-year-old child, but it did tend to wear on me, especially time after time.

My relationships with my friends have changed dramatically. We tend to be much more action-oriented in our activities (like biking, skiing, swimming, playing, etc.) as opposed to staying home and watching movies or other passive activities. I have a number of friends who accepted me for who I was when I was fat, *but* the relationships are much more vital and stimulating now that we can add a physical component to the mix.

With my family, the changes have been particularly profound. I have four kids (Brianne, 14; Andy, 12; Christian, 12; and Molly, 10). All of them were worried about me and were used to having a dad who basically just sat around and hurt. Now we do all sorts of things together (camping, swimming, skiing, biking, playing, wrestling). In addition, I believe that my children are happier and feel more secure, now that they don't worry so much about my health. The physical aspects of our relationships now tend to open the door to better emotional connectivity and spiritual discussions. It just seems easier to talk about important life issues when we are skiing together at Winter Park, versus chatting while dad lies immobile in bed.

The change in my relationship with my wife, Sue, is almost indescribable. Sue has always cared for me, loved me, and given herself to me physically. However, it was sometimes obvious that she yearned to make love with a husband of more normal proportions. I love how we can now hug and snuggle without my fat getting in the way! And, like my kids, I sense that Sue feels much more secure with a husband who is healthy and active and likely to be around for a long, long time.

Would I do it again? This is a tough decision for anyone, and I respect the fact that each person has to work through the issues. For me however, the short answer is *yes, I absolutely would do it again.* I have my life back. It has not been an easy road, but I finally have a tool that works in my battle against being overweight.

Beyond losing weight, though, I've had to learn how to struggle through pain and emotions without reaching for food or other negative things. This has been a bigger struggle for me than I anticipated. In hindsight, I would have spent more time getting ready for postsurgery life. Relearning to fill my life with positive replacements like my faith, family, fellowship, exercise, and rest has been a challenge. However, I am *so glad* that I am finally learning how to do this!

Here are the trade-offs that I made in having weight loss surgery.

What I Got:

- I got rid of my intolerable back pain, without the monthly spinal injections, OxyContin, narcotics, or back surgery.

- Within two months of my weight loss surgery, my joint pain also disappeared (preceded by the many thousands of dollars that I spent trying to figure out why I had so much joint pain in the first place).

- During that same time frame, my depression also lifted, after fifteen years of oppressing my spirits and limiting my life.

- Within two weeks of my gastric bypass, both my migraines and my sleep apnea were gone too. How wonderful and liberating it is to sleep without my CPAP machine!

- My blood pressure is now normal (110/70, down from 135/98), and my blood sugar levels and triglycerides are completely normal.

- These are just some of the more dramatic medical improvements in my life. Virtually every other aspect of my life is better too. My sex life is better. I sleep less, and enjoy more time to *do life!* People don't stare at me anymore. I can shop for my clothes anywhere, off the rack (with my size 34 waist). I am infused with energy.

- My lowest post-WLS weight was 157 (August 2003); today I've stabilized at a healthy (and very fit) 175 pounds (down 157 pounds from my highest pre-op weight).

What I've Given Up:

- I was very tired for the first 5–6 weeks after my surgery, but with time, the fatigue was replaced with more energy than I knew what to do with.

- I still experience some constipation.

- I will need to take extra vitamins and minerals every day for the rest of my life (because the gastric bypass results in malabsorption—my body doesn't absorb all of the nutrition in the food I consume). This is only a slight annoyance, but it is important to remember for long-term health.

- I've had to change my fundamental relationship with food from using it as a drug to using it as fuel, and to meet my emotional needs by replacement behaviors (such as exercising) and replacement tools (such as my faith).

- I continue to experience hanging folds of skin that were once filled with fat, although sound nutrition, vitamins, and exercise have helped to minimize the problem.

Before considering weight loss surgery, it's important to understand both the potential risks and rewards. Read about different WLS procedures. Make absolutely sure to choose a trained and experienced bariatric surgeon with a track record of success—one who provides a comprehensive program of pre- and postoperative care. Run away from providers who promise fantastic results and instant happiness.

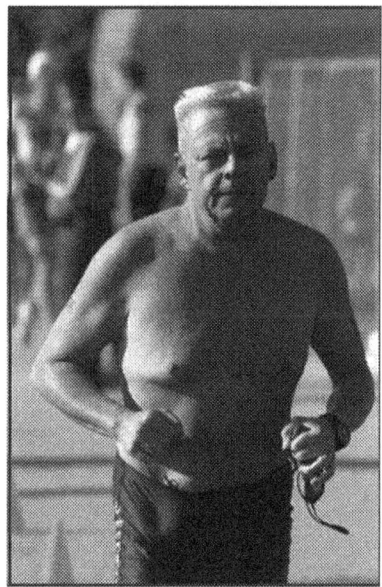

Weight loss surgery can be a wonderful tool to lose weight, but it is not a guarantee of a happy life. My happiness and joy in life come from doing the hard work of developing my faith, learning to love people with courage, and learning to enjoy life without stuffing something into my mouth! I used that first year post-op as an excellent season to learn and grow as a person.

11

It's All About Me!

by
Cindy Michaud

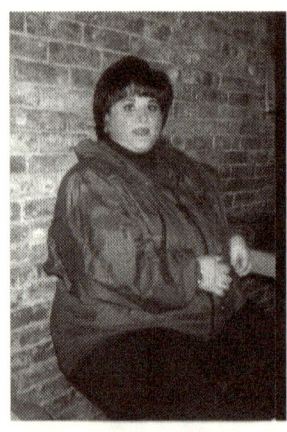

I could not remember a time when I wasn't heavy. I do remember seeing pictures of me when I was little, and although I was small, I almost always had food in my hand. It was a running joke; I could devour a whole sandwich before I was a year old. When I was about five, my aunt and uncle took my sisters, my cousins, and me to the beach. I never left the cooler. With a face covered with peanut butter and jelly, I looked at my uncle and said "Uncle Teddy, I am starving. I haven't eaten anything all day." He quickly picked me up, laughed, and fed my little peanut butter and jelly face. To this day, my uncle still asks me if I want a PB & J sandwich!

Between the ages of seven and eight, I doubled from a size 7 to a size 14. Growing up in an Italian family—where our social settings were *always* focused around food—it was no wonder that my once-petite frame eventually turned into that of an overweight child.

I remember times when my father would argue with my Nana, saying "Ma, stop feeding her; she's had enough!" I believe that my grandmother was just trying to show her love for me with her food. And I know that I was telling her just how much I loved her back by eating every morsel offered.

Everyone seemed to blame my emotional eating for my weight problem, and yet I really could not find a specific emotion that caused me to overeat. I just loved to eat. And for me, being social meant stuffing myself with food.

During my family gatherings, everyone passed around the pasta bowl and meatballs and told the others about their day. This is how we connected. Every Sunday was an *event*. We all gathered to eat at Nana's house. If you said you weren't hungry, it was as if it were a sin. And we all know that little Italian Catholic girls do not sin. To this day I have had to learn that I don't have to tie food to socializing with those I love.

I grew up with two sisters and two brothers. None were overweight. So for my teen years of early obesity, I really did not have anyone who could relate to how I felt. My sister Chrissy was one of the hardest on me. She couldn't understand how I could let myself get so big. She badgered me about my size. I would tease her about being skinny, and she screamed back that I was a "fat pig." These ugly exchanges still echo in my memory. (It wasn't until much later in my life that I began to understand that being too thin was as much of a struggle for her as my excess weight was for me.)

By the time I was a junior in high school I weighed 240 pounds. However, I was the *funny girl*, the one who always wore a smile on her face. I was intent on proving that I did not need to change my outside to be accepted. I *was* accepted, but mainly as the *big girl*. We all knew by junior year that the tantalizing, thrilling promise of proms lay just ahead. I was finally realizing that I would really like to be the one that got noticed, invited, and courted—not just known as the *funny big girl*.

So many times I heard, "Cindy, you have such a beautiful face," always followed by "if you could just lose a little weight." I wanted the skinny body to go with that pretty face. I think it was then when I really started down the disappointing path of an endless series of futile diets.

My first serious weight loss program was NutriSystem. This was going to be my saving grace! All my food was planned and required no cooking. All I had to do was add water to my pizza sauce. My Nana would have had a heart attack if she saw me prepare and eat that for dinner. But the weight started coming off.

However, not satisfied with a mere 2–3 pounds of weight loss per week, I started making my weekly food allocation last two weeks, then three weeks, and then even longer. I quickly lost over 100 pounds, but obviously not the healthy way. I was young and naïve. I thought the whole reason I had to be thin was to look good—not to be healthy.

When the thrill of that plan faded, I eventually tried the next fad diet that worked for everyone else (but not for me). I invariably ended up gaining back all the weight I had lost, plus more.

This was the start of a long and vicious circle of failed diets. Inevitably, my repeated compulsive dieting and subsequent failure became one of the root causes of my continuing, and worsening, obesity. This once confident adolescent teen swallowed societal pressures, expectations, and promises and bought into the misguided beliefs and misconceptions about body image. It's taken me decades to correct my misperceptions and stinking thinking.

I don't want you to think that being obese ruled my everyday life. It didn't. Even though I was heavy, I always took care of myself. I never left the house without looking my best, and I continued to live what I believed to be a successful life.

I had several good relationships before my marriage. The one I remember most was the one right before I met my future husband. He said that my weight made him "feel even smaller" than he actually was. He was probably the smallest guy I had ever dated, but *I* wasn't shallow, and I looked past *his* issues of size because I really cared about him.

This was the first time I actually heard a man tell me that my weight bothered him. I knew that it bothered *me*, but didn't know—before this—that it bothered *him*. I told him that it was his problem and went on with my life, but that experience bothered me for a long time as it was the first time I didn't feel accepted in a relationship for who I really was.

When I was least expecting it, I met my husband, Tony. I met him when I weighed 275 pounds, and I was only twenty-three years old. At the time, I wasn't really seeking a significant other. I felt self-assured and complete. I knew, in my heart of hearts, that when someone truly accepted and loved me for my essence, I would be enough, no matter what I weighed or how I looked.

When Tony looked at me, he looked past my weight, and saw the whole package. I was never a size to him. I was a person—a person he loved. He always told me it was my strength and perseverance that first attracted him to me. We are now approaching our seventh anniversary, and have been blessed with two healthy, beautiful children (Trevor and Camryn).

Tony and my children were my three biggest factors in wanting to be healthy. I wanted to live long enough to see my children get married, have children, and be a part of their lives. Every day I was realizing that my excess weight was reducing my chances to fulfill this ultimate life goal.

As I mentioned before, my sister Chrissy was not my biggest fan as a fat woman. We had moved past the times of teasing each other about our weights, but she was still adamant that I do something about it. She expressed her very real fear that my weight would catch up with me, and she was afraid of my dying prematurely. I knew she was speaking from her heart, but her accusations often made me feel defensive. I continued to insist that I was happy with who I was and didn't need to change. I knew secretly, deep inside, that she was right. But how could I admit that to her? That would be like losing the battle and admitting failure and defeat. I convinced myself that I could go on living heavy, no matter how society judged or labeled me, and that I could still be healthy. I was *so* wrong, and in the months ahead, I discovered that I would lose our lifelong argument.

In February 2003 I hit my all-time heaviest weight—330 pounds—even after all those years of attempting one diet after another. I finally found the one doctor with whom I felt comfortable enough to share my most personal issues. I had always tried to avoid seeing doctors, because I would have to disrobe and expose my fat self.

It was both funny and terribly ironic. I found that most doctors would look at me and say, "Cindy, your problems are due to your being so over-weight." It was so ludicrous. They talked and acted as if I didn't already know that I was fat, as if they had just diagnosed me with a new condition. Deep down inside, I wanted my doctor to confront me with reality and my options. I knew that I was slowly killing myself, albeit with a smile on my face, and on some deep level I wanted my denial to be challenged by my doctor.

It was a cool, brisk New England day in February 2003 that changed my life forever! At age twenty-nine, after a commute home to pick up my children, I stepped out of my van and collapsed in the driveway of my daycare provider. As I lay motionless and helpless on the frozen driveway, my children watched from the window in a state of total terror. I was quickly rushed to the hospital and, after a full night of tests, I was diagnosed with diabetes.

My blood sugar had dropped to 30 because I thought, in my insanity, that going all day without eating was my best way to lose weight. My doctor looked at me and said, "Cindy, if you don't do something about your weight, you are going to die as a very young woman." I sat there in total desperation, wondering what I was going to say to my beloved children. I could no longer deny the truth. My morbid obesity was jeopardizing the quality—and even the continuation—of my life. Was I finally ready to actually *do* something about it?

It broke my heart the next day when my five-year-old son, Trevor, asked me, "Mom, did you die yesterday?" Grasping for an appropriate answer, I replied, "You know, Trevor, part of me did. And I *am* going to do something about it…we are going to be all right!" It was then that I realized I owed my children so much more. I realized that I owed *me* so much more!

I started my new life as a morbidly obese diabetic. The choice was mine. Would I be paralyzed by my fear, guilt, and shame, or would I move into action? I had been heavy my whole life, and honestly, my weight felt like an integral part of me. I liked who I was, but I could no longer deny that my life-long disease of obesity had finally caught up to me. My health crisis was banging insistently on my door, and I had no choice but to answer the call and face my dilemma head on.

I logged on to the computer, not even knowing what I was looking for, and stumbled on the Web site for Dr. Aslam. He offered an incredible amount of information and had a comprehensive support system in place for the surgery he performed, called *gastric bypass surgery*. I started asking questions. I nervously typed in my weight and height to find out my BMI (body mass index). (Previously, I would have thought BMI was a brand of car.) I was startled to find that my BMI was 59—characterized as "Super Morbidly Obese." I looked over at Tony, with fear in my eyes, and he said the words I needed to hear: "What will it hurt to explore this option?" I knew that this was an avenue I *had* to explore. I started down my WLS path.

When I set a new goal, I complete it. My pursuit of weight loss surgery information became my new quest. Tony and I went to WLS support group meetings. I talked with other patients and probed them with my endless questions. I constantly heard people discussing their "relationship with food" and their "emotional eating habits." I had never before considered food as my emotional band-aid. Was it? I desperately needed to figure this all out before I was ready to consider undergoing this drastic medical procedure of gastric bypass surgery.

Before I could even be considered for surgery, I was required to meet with a nutritionist and a psychiatrist and to attend at least two of my bariatric surgeon's support group meetings. These events are what helped me figure things out and get the answers I needed.

Tony accompanied me to almost every meeting. I think sometimes we tend to forget or neglect those who aren't having the surgery, but who provide us with an indispensable support system throughout the process. My weight loss surgery was going to mean major changes for Tony, not just me.

Together, we were finally able to realize and acknowledge that even though my stomach would be smaller, I would still be the same person. Somehow, that made it okay. My choice was made. I would have weight loss surgery!

I set about the task of educating my family. They were worried, but as I shared the information I had gathered, they came to understand that this was a chance for a new beginning for me.

My father and I had always been close, but never really "mushy." When he visited me in the hospital after I was diagnosed with diabetes, it was the first time he really showed how he felt about my weight problem. It was agony for me to see the tears in his eyes, and to hear the concern in his voice. I knew that he loved me—big or small—but I could tell how worried he was. All he knew about gastric bypass were the horror stories of complications, and worse, the deaths. But he had faith in me and supported my decision.

I underwent my gastric bypass surgery on April 28, 2003. This was one of the best choices I have ever made in my life! I am 17 months post-op now, and I have lost 170 pounds to this date.

I was terrified on the morning of my surgery as I lay on the operating table. I had just signed my name on the dotted line of my living will. Writing down my wishes if I did not survive the surgery was the hardest thing I had ever done. I wrote letters to my family letting them know this was my choice, my future, my life. I was willing to risk the surgery since the risks of continuing to live as a morbidly obese woman were even worse than the possibilities of complications or even dying on the table.

My hospital stay was short, and my complications were few. Physically, I felt little pain. Emotionally, however, I was devastated. No matter how much I had prepared for my surgery, I still mourned the loss of food. My life-long love affair with food was now over, forever. I must have watched the Food Channel every day for weeks during my recuperation, just imagining how the food would taste.

Then suddenly, one day, something clicked and everything fell into place for me. I literally leaped off my pity pot, and realized that I had been given a precious second chance, a gift that I could never repay. I realized that *now* was the time to get my life back.

I went back to work after four weeks. For me, returning to my daily routine helped with my recovery. I did not want to sit idle at home and dwell on the changes I had undergone. I just wanted to get on with the rest of my life.

The thing that helped me most was that I completely understood that this WLS was *only a tool*. My primary challenge was to find the best way to effectively and productively utilize this tool. Learning how to deal with my emotions turned out to be another vital coping skill. The surgery gave me the confidence I needed to deal with the feelings that had, unconsciously, driven me to overeat.

As my weight started coming off, I was able to become much more mobile, and the exercise greatly accelerated my weight loss. Before my surgery, my "exercise" involved standing up to grab the Ben & Jerry's from the fridge. Now exercise is a vital, treasured, and consistent part of my daily routine. I think my son, Trevor, just about fainted when I threatened to get off the couch when he was doing something wrong, and I did get up to stop him. The look on his face was priceless. Things had changed in our household!

My surgery has liberated me from the pressures, pain, and pangs of hunger. Once these disappeared, I learned that I could actually stop eating when I was full. My presurgical stomach size never allowed me the satiety of fullness. And in the months ahead, I paired my knowledge of healthy eating with my fullness and moved on to live a healthy life.

During my recovery and weight loss, I realized there were so many topics, tips, and issues I wanted to discuss with others who could really understand. Consequently, I started my own support group, called "It's All About ME!" That name says it all!

In October 2003, our group teamed up with the American Diabetes Association to conduct a Walk-a-Thon. We walked for our own health, as well as to raise money for a cause that is very important to me. (My mom still suffers from diabetes, and although her disease was not a product of any obesity.) When I walked for the American Diabetes Association, I was *diabetes free!* No more medication! That was one of my proudest moments, and I owe it all to my weight loss surgery, to my commitment and determination, and to my support system.

This is my time to become a little selfish and to care as much about myself as I've always cared about and for others. It is my time to feel beautiful, both inside and out! I am so proud of who I was, who I am, and who I will always be.

I did *not* have this surgery to take the easy way out. I have had to learn to address things about myself that I didn't even want to know, and I've had to acknowledge and deal with my feelings. I used to fantasize about the "miracle cure" for my obesity. I know now that there's no cure—that achieving and maintaining my weight loss requires hard work and determination. Exercise and healthy eating will always remain essential components of my life and my weight loss success.

I never want to forget the old, heavy me. I still love her dearly. It's just that now I equally love and cherish the *new* Cindy, who can live a fuller, healthier, more active, and longer life because of the decisions I have made and the actions I have taken.

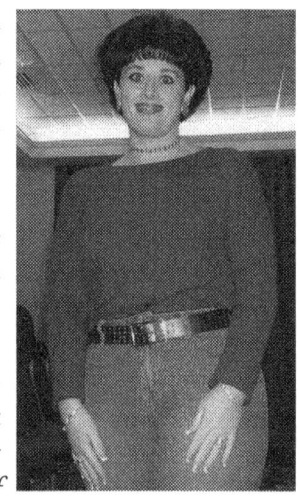

Nothing is going to keep me from my goals! Everyday is a chance for me to stop being on the sidelines. Before my surgery, my goals always seemed to be something I talked about. Now I achieve them!

I thank God everyday that I have had the courage, and the support, to take this WLS journey. It has not been easy. I have had to overcome many obstacles along the way. But today, I am a *woman of strength* whose future is no longer dictated or defined by fear, failure, or despair!

Afterword:

A Postscript
from Glenn's Wife

A Postscript from Glenn's Wife
or
The Blessings of Two Years in a Trim and Active Body

I'm Kari Goldberg, Glenn's wife, writing with sad news. On December 19, 2004, Glenn suddenly died, doing what he loved most—walking on one of the beautiful trails here in the Pacific Northwest. He was happy, seemingly healthy, and enjoying being with a friend. Literally in the middle of a joke, he paused for a moment and then dropped dead. This was a shock to all who knew him either in person or via the Web.

One of the first thoughts I had was whether weight loss surgery had anything to do with this. Is this somehow our fault for making that choice? I now have the autopsy report and can answer these questions with a very resounding *no*!

Let me explain. Glenn died of a massive heart attack. It was quick and painless. He did not suffer. What they found was that three of the four vessels attached to the heart were 80–90% blocked! I reminded our doctor that Glenn had a treadmill test in March 2004, after which the doctors said that Glenn "had the heart of an athlete." He was so proud of that. Why wasn't this blockage noticed? The doctor said that the machine is not 100% foolproof, and that it probably did not pick up the problem because Glenn was so fit from having lost all the weight and his daily walking.

Now, here's the kicker. First, I need to tell you that Glenn was always very good about going in to the doctor for his annual check-up. Apparently, sometime between the last physical and December 19, 2004, he had developed a rapidly developing form of acute leukemia! It was in all his organs and blood. He had no symptoms.

What this means to me is that it was truly Glenn's time to die. He was either going to die in this fast, painless way or in a longer, chemo-filled, painful way. I think Glenn (or the Universe) chose wisely.

I specifically asked the doctor if the weight loss surgery was in *any* way responsible for Glenn's death. He asked me when his surgery was—"October 2002" was my response. He said, "Well, given what we know now in terms of vessel blockages, without the surgery in October 2002, he probably would have been dead by January 2003!" The WLS gave him two years to have a trim body, to put food in proper perspective, and to travel to England, the Bahamas, Florida, and North Carolina. He was able to recently see his family and friends. He saw our daughter's first professional place of employment. He played in the Atlantic Ocean. He was filled with gratitude.

What I had been feeling was that Glenn was robbed of his life. What I felt after hearing the autopsy report was that it was truly Glenn's time to die (for whatever reason). I'm still deep in sorrow but calmer in my heart.

Glenn was an organ donor, and therefore continues to give to others. His corneas have allowed two people to see again. Some of his bone was used to help with orthopedic reconstruction and dental surgery. And what would have pleased him most of all is that his excess skin (that he hated so much and wanted the surgery to remove but we could not afford it) was removed and will be used to help burn victims heal. I am very proud of this man.

If Glenn were standing in front of me right now and we were somehow able to see all that happened between his surgery and his death, I have absolutely no doubt that he would choose the exact same path. Weight loss surgery gave him a much fuller, more complete life. And he enjoyed every second of it.

Coping with death is always hard, but it is my strong hope that you will not connect Glenn's writings (and WLS) with his death. It was just his time to go. I feel blessed to have had twenty-five years with such a passionate, caring, and self-aware human being. It was my privilege and honor.

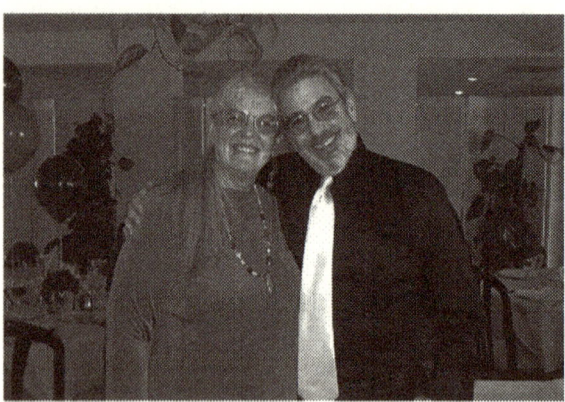

Kari and Glenn Goldberg, November 20, 2004

978-0-595-37968-2
0-595-37968-0